RENEE IN CANCERLAND

Renee Sendelbach

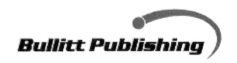

ISBN-13 978-0-9858947-5-7

First Edition

RENEE IN CANCERLAND

Copyright © 2014 by Renee Sendelbach

Published by Bullitt Publishing, LLC

www.bullittpublishing.com

PRINTED IN U.S.A.

Cover design by: Renee Sendelbach

A note to my readers:

I have gone back and forth with myself on how to actually write this whole book because let's call a spade a spade: this IS my first rodeo.

I have gotten advice on how I should approach writing this book, which tense to write in, but when I look at me - at who I really am, I knew from the beginning I wouldn't be taking any of that advice.

With that being said, please know I realize this book isn't 100% perfect. In all honesty, I don't want it to be perfect. I am not in any way perfect, so why would something I write be perfect? I don't have a grammar book sitting next to me to look up run-on sentences (even if I did, I wouldn't use it), I don't have an English degree — I just have many life lessons I want to pass on to you.

This is me.

I want you to hear my voice telling you this story and in order to do that, I have to write like I talk...sometimes long-winded, sometimes short and messy, sometimes short and sweet, or sometimes no point is ever really made. But I promise you this, this is all from my heart.

With that being said, I never intended to write a book. Well, I guess I never intended to have Stage IV breast cancer either. This book has been six years in the making.

At 30 years old, I thought I was going to be raising children, strengthening my marriage and doing my part in the community. However, at 30, I found myself in a whole new world...cancerland.

Yep, I was thrown the cancer card.

I am writing this now to help get it out of me and relive it in a way that I can look back on with a new perspective. I hope by doing this, it will no longer sneak up and attack me with dread, fear and pain that hits so hard at such unexpected times.

Before I get into all that, let's get the messy details out of the way:

30 years old

My baby boy just turned 1 year old.

I felt the lump

Breast cancer

Chemo, surgery, radiation then clean and clear!

Life went on

32 years old

Routine scan

Heard the most heart breaking words – Stage IV Breast Cancer

I wish it were really that quick and easy as the nice little outline I wrote for you, but it is so far from that. So, SO far from that.

It has taken me many years of processing what Stage IV cancer means, treatable but not curable. Those words, "treatable but not curable" haunted me for years.

These words are devastating, the journey terrifying. There is no way to sugarcoat it so I won't even try, but hopefully through my experiences you will see, it doesn't have to be the end.

This has been the longest, hardest, most heartbreaking yet fulfilling journey I could have never imagined as my life. I am putting this out it into the world to help others see what is possible and what really matters through it all. Not just through cancer, but through life.

It is hard to comprehend the blessings that others have brought me; the only way to serve these blessings is to share them with others. It is my prayer that you draw some strength and wisdom from this book and my journey and know that there is more to life beyond the initial cancer diagnosis.

I have met and been helped by so many people I can't ever begin to start a list to thank them all. They are all so appreciated and loved it is hard to comprehend at times.

My hope is that those who going through a hard time can draw some strength and wisdom from my experiences and know that there is more to life beyond that initial blow that is so devastating …for me it was "cancer" but for you, could be anything.

With love,

Renee

Welcome to Renee In Cancerland...

List of characters

Family

Renee Sendelbach – the one with cancer

Eric Sendelbach – my husband

Ian – our son

Mom – my mom

Dad – my dad

Rachele – my sister

Mom & Dad S – Eric's parents

Erics's sisters

Doctors:

Dr. H – Dr. Beth Hellerstadt, Renee's oncologist

Dr. Cutie – Dr. James Waldron, Renee's brain surgeon

Groves – Dr. Mortie Groves, Renee's brain oncologist

Shinebine - Dr. Courtney Shinebine, Renee's radiation oncologist

Dr. N – breast surgeon who gave me news

Anybody else named in the book is a close friend of mine.

2008

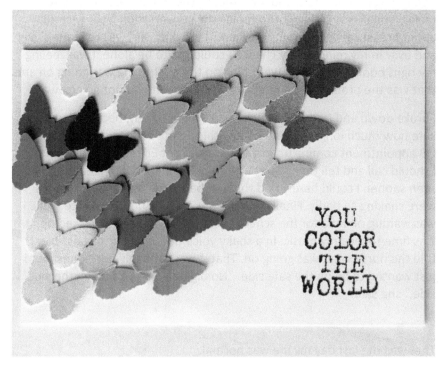

I felt it for the first time just a few days after my baby boy's first birthday.

The lump - August, 2008

The hot water was pounding onto my back as I stood there in disbelief telling myself this had to be my imagination. There is no way this lump I am feeling was real and if it is real, it must have something to do with hormones. After all, my body was just now returning to normal after having Ian, breastfeeding for 4 months and my period returning. My mind raced back to just yesterday while I was at work talking to my friends about breast cancer and how it seems to be all over the place these days. We all were asking each other if we each did self-breast exams.

No, was the answer all around. I fought with myself for a few seconds before I went in for a second feel. Yup, it was still there. My mind was racing while I was trying not to replay the conversation from yesterday about breast cancer in young women. "I am only 30," was repeating over and over in my mind. Every chance I could get to be alone, I was feeling my right boob to see what was going on there. Nothing was going on and that was the problem. The lump was still there. It was not going away.

I broke down and told my husband, Eric, the next day, because I wasn't sure how much longer I could handle this on my own. I had my yearly OB appointment coming up in a few weeks, but Eric told me he thought I should call and tell them what was going on and ask if I needed to be seen sooner. I could barely find the number in my phone as my hands were shaking so badly. Finally, I found it. I actually hung up twice while I was waiting on hold for the scheduler. Once the other side picked up, it was time to face my music. In a shaky voice but as calmly as possible, I told the nurse what was going on. That it was probably hormones, but I just wanted to be on the safe side. "No big deal but let's be on the safe side," she said.

That was the last day my life was normal.

The first 24 hours - September 10, 2008

The call came in a little after 2:00 p.m., as I was sitting in my office at work. "Renee, hi this is Dr. N. I have your results from the biopsy. I am so sorry to tell you that it is cancer."

My heart stopped right then. My knees buckled as I had to brace myself on my desk. I didn't make a sound for a few seconds, until I willed myself to breathe. Then all the sounds came out at once as a crying scream. I kept saying No! No, this can't be. NO! I knew in my heart that when I had the biopsy it was going to be something but I sure didn't think it was going to be this. I mean, come on, I was THIRTY years old, had a precious baby boy, a wonderful husband, family and friends that were the best. How could I get cancer??

When I heard the words, I shut down. My manager and co-workers were there by my side. My manager, Mary, talked to the doctor on the phone while my co-workers packed my stuff up. They hugged me tight while I collapsed in their arms and sobbed, asking over and over how can this be happening, how can this actually be happening? The look of shock on their faces completely expressed the feelings that were clenching my throat. I didn't know what to say or do. Mary arranged for them to drive me home and wait with me at home until Eric got home from work.

When I called Eric to come home, he knew something big was wrong. Not long after my call to him, he was home – standing there in our living room.

In my mind, it wasn't real until I spoke the words to him. "It isn't good. I have cancer," I cried.

Cancer, what a crazy word, six letters that will change your life forever. It is a word we all talk about but when it comes to telling a loved one you have it, it doesn't come as easily. I am not sure when my co-workers left, but all of a sudden Eric and I were there by ourselves; left to hug each other and cry out all the tears we had at that time.

At some point I snapped out of it because I wanted to go pick up Ian from daycare. I just wanted to hug him and hold him as tight as I could. I wanted to be reminded why I was so ready to fight: his laugh, his smile, his love for me, and his love for his daddy. Eric and I went to pick up Ian from daycare to take him to the pool. Something about watching him swim, having him give me sweet wet hugs and kisses, listening to him laugh, all of it let me forget the whole mess for those sweet moments.

Until bath time…While Ian was in the bath I had the sensation that I was floating above us in the bathroom, looking down on us in the bathroom. This came in waves. It was the most surreal thing I have ever experienced. I was at peace while I was floating, but I knew it wasn't real.

I held Ian a long time that night even after he fell asleep.

I held him and cried.

I cried for him, for him having to have a mom with cancer.

I cried because I didn't know how long he would have a mommy.

I cried because I wanted his life to be perfect and mommy having cancer wasn't perfect.

It was time though – I had to do something.

I called my mom first. She wasn't even able to say hello before I broke down into sobs. Gut wrenching sobs. Sobs I was sure would eventually take my breath away. I was so sure if I told my mom that she could somehow magically make it all go away. I couldn't get full sentences out, but between my sobs and the few words I got out, her world was now free falling too. I had just told her that her 30 year old baby girl had breast cancer. That was all I could say – I have cancer. She kept repeating that it will be ok, and we will get through this, over and over. I know she was telling herself that as much as she was telling me.

Eric held me.

I held him.

We held each other.

We held each other in the uncertainty of where our lives were heading.

We held each other for better or worse.

We didn't know which way was up or down, but we vowed to each other we would do this.

We vowed that day that we would do this together; whatever this turned out to be.

I still had to tell my dad, sister, in-laws and friends. I called my sister first, but she wasn't home so my brother-in-law got the news. I can honestly say this was one time he wasn't able to say something smartass back to me. Hey, I had to take what I could at this point.

Next on the list was my dad. My dad is a man of very few words and when I told him, he was a man of even fewer words. He wanted to know if this was 100% correct. How were they sure? I heard the choked back cry as he told me he loved me. I was wrecked with emotion. My heart hurt more than I could ever imagine. It hurt because I knew I was making other's hearts hurt.

Eric and I sat together the whole night on the couch holding on to each other. Even during the phone calls, we sat, held each other and cried. My sister called me back. Part of me was hoping she wouldn't call back so I could continue to hide from the truth. As soon as I answered we both just cried. We went over everything I knew, and then I was done. I had nothing left to give. I had no more energy to continue this path of destruction. I made Eric call his mom, and she took on the daunting task of telling the rest of family. I was still not sure I had processed this. I got waves of tears, then just laughed about it, then a surreal feeling of what in the hell was going on and where was I? That was what I was afraid of – Where am I?

Just Breathe – September 17, 2008

Just breathe was all I could tell myself while sitting waiting to be called back to meet my new oncologist. A month ago I didn't even know what an oncologist was, and now I had one. I sat there looking at the clientele and I felt like a purple alien. I felt like people wouldn't look at me. Maybe they knew something I didn't know.

Maybe they were afraid I was there by myself and I would leach on to them to hold me up.

Maybe it was all part of my imagination.

I am pretty sure no one really cared that I was sitting there, but I felt like people were asking themselves, "is she waiting for her mom?" Nope! I am here for me. Please look away; there is nothing to see here is what I wanted to shout out in the waiting room. Of course I didn't though - I rarely say anything I really want to out loud if it isn't something halfway nice. Instead I said a lot of prayers in my head, but no spoken words. I watched a few people walked in for a class. I think it was a class on chemo, but I am not 100% sure as I couldn't hear all the details. I was trying to look like I was reading a book and not fall out of my chair as I leaned further and further over to hear more of what everyone was saying. I was sure this was a class I would eventually have to take.

After filling out yet more paper work, I tried to actually read this time. That didn't get me too far as I reread the same paragraph at least five times and still had no idea what I just read. "Renee Sendelbach," I heard the lady say. Oh wow, she got the last name correct was what I thought to myself. I let the front desk know that Eric was on his way and to please let him back. I had to get my height and weight again. I really don't know why they wouldn't let me tell them this information; probably because I would lie. I was trying to take it all in on my way back to my room. There were so many rooms with the doors closed. Did that mean other patients were in those rooms as well? There I was sitting in this room looking at the artwork and family pictures on the walls. Pictures I was guessing were of Dr. H and her family. All the while I was waiting for someone, anyone to come in. Eric, the doctor, the nurse, someone to come in, clap their hands in the air and tell me it was time to wake up and go home. This bad dream was over and I handled it all pretty well.

No one ever came in to tell me that.

Dr. H, my oncologist, came in and started going over the very basic stuff until Eric got there. I was really not sure what all she said. I did think to myself that she was my girl. She stomped around her office in killer five-inch heals that you could hear coming down the hall a few doors away. She was a tiny little thing, but something with her and I clicked right away. Eric arrived a few minutes later and now was the time to get to the meat of the matter. What were my options from here? Dr. H was great. She was very to the point but in a kind way. She didn't beat around the bush, which is fine with me. I was at the point with all this that I just needed to know what we were dealing with so I knew what all was on the table.

Here was what we now knew: I had my blood drawn to have it tested for a DNA mutation. If it came back positive, there was a high likely hood that I would have a double mastectomy and possibly my ovaries taken out. The reason behind this was if I did have the mutation, there was a 90% chance of breast cancer recurrence and 96% chance of ovarian cancer. All I could think at this point, was WTF??? Who started talking about ovarian cancer? I was here for breast cancer. If I didn't have this mutation, we would think about starting chemo before doing the lumpectomy. As Dr. H kindly put it, she was afraid of the "divot" my breast would have if we did the lumpectomy right in the beginning with the tumor being as large as it was. If it was estrogen driven, I would be on medicine to suck the estrogen out of my body. Oh, I was sure that would be an interesting hormonal rollercoaster for everyone to deal with! There was another slew of options that we could have been looking at, but before I could pick out of the black box and pull out "my prize" of what I actually did have, I had to become a human lab rat. I was getting a PT scan and bone scan tomorrow. She said she had no reason to believe it was elsewhere in my body but wanted to get all the facts before starting anything. Then sometime next week I would get a biopsy of the cancer.

And then WHAM, we were hit with something that was in the back of my mind but I had not talked about it out loud. She was talking about seeing a fertility doctor. I was so confused at this point. All I could think to myself was why would I need to see a fertility doctor? We got pregnant so easily the first time around. Now with cancer in the mix, depending on what type of cancer I had, there was a possibility my baby makin' days were over. Sitting there trying to process all of this, nothing made much sense.

I am not sure if I am in denial or what, but I didn't cry - I was all cried out. And when I did talk about it, I felt like I talked about it so matter of fact. I was sure one day it would hit me like a brick wall what was going on and that no, I was not in a 2 week long bad dream. I was in the middle of my new reality and I would deal with it like I had dealt with anything else in life. Look it in the eyes and deal with it.

A fish out of water – September 18, 2008

I felt like a fish out of water. Well, I think that was how I felt. I was not real sure how a fish out of water really felt. But if the feeling was difficulty breathing and only focusing on getting back to the water, then yes. Yes that is how I felt. All I wanted right now was for us to go back to our drama free lives. We were so happy sans drama.

Just a few days ago, just a few short days ago, none of this was going on.

I had an appointment with my breast surgeon this morning.

That place was depressing.

For way too long, I sat half naked with a flimsy paper gown on, that had to be open to the front, the ac turned down to freezing and an IV stuck in my hand with a syringe taped down to my hand. This was all after the nurse who put my IV in missed the first stick of the IV in my arm and had to do it again in my hand. Really? Really? How do you fucking miss my vein? This is what you do all damn day, I wanted to yell. But I didn't. I didn't say anything out loud. I just prayed quietly in my heart hoping this somehow wasn't real.

Before the hurrah here, Eric and I already had a very rough morning. We went to the fertility specialist to talk with her nurse about our situation. As I said before, the hardest part for me from all this was the thought of not being able to have another baby. Again, we received so much information in such a little time frame. A time frame in which tears were shed and laughs occurred. I was not sure how to put into words how I felt about the possibility of me not being able to have another child. It wasn't that I didn't feel 100% complete with our family of three because I did. And I knew if Ian had to grow up without a brother or sister, he would be ok – he had a ton of little friends and cousins galore. It was just one of the hardest things to hear that I might not be able to give him a brother or sister. I couldn't imagine my life without my sister and I looked at my nieces and nephews and couldn't imagine them without the other.

So there we sat, with this chart of expenses in front of us and all I could think is how can we put a price on this decision? Price aside, I had to figure out what my odds were going to be for me to carry a baby. After a lengthy discussion with Eric, we were both in agreement that we didn't want a surrogate to carry our child. So, all this was going to ride on what type of cancer I had. If it was estrogen driven, I was fairly certain I would not be able to even carry a child. But then if it was a DNA type, I THOUGHT I would possibly be able to carry. And of course, no matter what type it was, a lot would depend on the chemo treatment I received and if it was going to throw me into early menopause. I might go through menopause before my mom. Nice, I guess I would be able to give her helpful advice.

No matter what we looked at, how we looked at it, I was certain this would be one of the most difficult decisions we would ever have to make. I just kept thinking, what if she tells me, you won't be able to carry a child and then by some huge miracle, I would be able to but we didn't freeze any embryos? Or what if we freeze 10 embryos and then I can't carry a child? All I can think about is what if I am leaving 10 kids frozen in time? What are my beliefs here and how do I figure them out in 24 hours? And I just didn't think there was anyone who could help me decide this. Only my heart and my heart was so torn right then I didn't know what to think. All I knew was that we had to decide soon. Like in two days soon. I either started the egg harvesting medicine now or I didn't.

There were so many balls in the air for Eric and I to try to catch, exam and throw back up to keep the juggling act going.

This had been a hard day.

The odds – September 21, 2008
I would like to think I don't live completely by the odds, but I guess to some extent I do.

What are the odds it will rain today?

What are the odds I will make it to work on time if I leave 5 minutes late?

What are the odds I will win the lottery today? (Not very good!)

After looking into our hearts, thinking through every possible scenario inside and out, deciding where I stood ethically, I looked at our odds. We are going with the odds in my favor - 80% chance of me regaining normal periods after chemo is finished and 100% faith in God and our decision. We decided against the harvesting process for so many reasons.

My biggest reason for saying no to it was the fact I had no idea when life actually did begin. I know there are scientists out there that say the embryo isn't alive until it's producing blood on its own (or something like that - science really isn't my strong suit) and most religions believe it begins as early as the sperm meets the egg. No one really knows and we never will, but I wanted to do the right thing by me and the would-have-been embryos. I just couldn't imagine if life did begin at the embryo state, me having something to do with freezing however many embryos for however long - possibly forever.

Let me tell you, facing an ethical decision like this was so much harder living in the middle of it verses forming an opinion while standing on outside looking in. Everyone likes to sit on a high horse and say what they would or wouldn't do. But until you are in the situation, you never know what you will do. I was so emotionally vested in this. I could not see past the thought of I would be a horrible mother to Ian if I wasn't able to give him a sibling.

But then I had to remember back to when this all began (oh, a whole 10 days ago) and remember what I told myself, I will take this one day at a time. Because if I look at the whole picture, it will scare the living crap out of me. So, looking at today, I have to look out for my health first and foremost, get this shit taken care of. Then we will move on with the possibility of another child. Looking at it from this perspective really helped us make the decision. I have to be the best mother to Ian right now. He will forgive me if I didn't give him a sibling. He won't forgive me if I don't take care of myself. And it was crazy, once Eric and I both said no to each other, I felt peace in my heart and knew we made the right decision.

Smile. Yes please. Thank You – September 22, 2008

That string of words looks so simple when read from paper. But saying them, learning to really say them was something I have a hard time with...a really hard time. Don't get me wrong, I smile all the time. I give genuine smiles from my heart to people all day long. My heart has no choice but to smile, it just happens. I always said thank you to whomever was helping me do whatever it is they were helping me with. Be it my hubby for fixing my computer issues, my friends for picking up the slack in my mommy duties, my nurses at chemo or to my waiter for his service. But when it comes to accepting help from those outside of my familiar circle, these words didn't come easy and sometimes they didn't come at all. Instead, I smiled and dug a little deeper every time to come up with, "I am fine."

I am fiercely independent and even more stubborn. Thanks to my mom raising me to know I can do anything on my own, I have taken that with me throughout my life. But I was beginning to wonder –was this the best way to approach life? I was beginning to realize that I did need help. I had always needed help. I had always felt guilty about needing help. Oh guilt, that was a fun emotion to try to dissect. I obviously hadn't gotten all the way through that! One of my goals to learn while on this journey was that people didn't mind doing things to help me in whatever form I needed them. In fact they wanted to. Just like I want to do so much for others; and most of all, when they offer to help, it was sincere and they weren't just saying it to be polite. Little unknown fact about me: I had a

therapist once ask me if I was Catholic because of all the guilt I carried
around.

Port-a-what? – September 23, 2008

Everything went well today. I had a porta-cath installed in my chest wall
and a core biopsy of the tumor. All this happened while I was taking a
nice IV induced nap. I know it is bad to say, but that second right when
the IV drug hits and my mind went to that place where none of this was
real was a great moment. But I was smart enough to know not to mess
with that shit outside of medical purposes. That was my happy cocktail.
My happy cocktail made me remember nothing from the surgery and
wake up still feeling good. I told Eric while I was sobering up, I felt like
I had a night out that I would tell my friends I would be right back but
instead go to bed and pass out! HA, we sure hadn't had one of those
nights in well over two years. Unfortunately once the cocktail wore off,
the pain came on pretty intense.

My left shoulder was still incredibly sore from where they put in the
port. I didn't realize it, but the port was in my muscle. My doctor told
me to expect to be sore for about three to five days. And I couldn't lift
anything heavy so that meant lifting my 28 pound love bug was out of
picture for a few days. Luckily Eric was awesome and would pick him up
from school and handle the nightly duties. This was the hardest part for
me, not being able to take care of our son. But, I had to remember, I was
taking care of him by taking care of myself.

Sit down, buckle up and hold on – September 30, 2008

This is going to be one heck of a ride. Today was surreal and I don't really
know if I have processed all this. I felt numb, pissed and scared shitless.
I really didn't ever want to feel pissed about having cancer but I did...still
do.

I am/was pissed at myself for letting myself believe this was somehow going to be easy.

I am/was pissed because I was told getting chemo was a BIG part of the plan. I had a plan damn it. Do you hear me God?? I HAD A PLAN. I was going to be able to skirt by this with no chemo, get a double mastectomy, get new boobs and call it good. Well, no new boobs for me and shit load of other things that were not in my plan. I have no control over any of it, none of it.

Now, I am scared out of my mind. I have no idea what chemo is going to be like. I have no idea what chemo is going to do to me. I have a lovely list of what it can do to me. I am too scared to read that list, so I threw it away. Hey, nothing like avoidance to get me through the day!? I have a list of what medicines I can take to help with nausea but there are some things I can't take medicine for like tiredness, taste buds changing, and hair loss. Now, I know I currently look cute with short hair, but am I going to look cute with NO hair? Will Ian look at me differently? Will Eric still think I was his beautiful wife? Will I stick out like a sore thumb no matter where I go? I fell like wearing a scarf will just scream CANCER. Hey, over here, I have cancer. I just didn't know. I just don't fucking know.

I am scared of the tiredness. I already feel bad for everything that I know Eric is going to have to take care of. I HATE not being able to pull my own weight and help him out. I am so worried about me not being be able to be the great mom to Ian I love being. As my doctor has told me twice now, I need to go ahead and get it in my head that I will not be winning any mother, wife, employee, friend of the year awards.

Nice. That was good to hear. The taste bud changing bit doesn't really bother me. I have always said if there was ever a time when I couldn't taste, I would eat chicken, rice and beans. Hey, I might be able to lose these 10 pounds I had been trying to lose forever!!

So I sat there to hear my pickings out of the big black box of cancer possibilities. I felt like I was waiting there for her to call bingo numbers out, except this wasn't a cash prize.

It wasn't any kind of prize.

It was my life being pulled out of this stupid box.

I am what they call triple negative. I am ER -, PR- and HER2-. How Eric explained it to me: this cancer in my body is NOT caused by estrogen, progesterone or HER2. Trip neg. is cancer that has been getting a lot of press lately due to them defining it by a lack of positive results. With the lack of any positive, they aren't real sure why the cancer occurs. The best guess is one little stubborn cell gets the wrong message and starts duplicating itself like it was someone important and now has caused havoc within my body. The good news here is that it could be treated with a variety of chemo cocktails whereas if it was ER+ or PR+ there were only a few cocktails to treat with.

I also found out, I was Stage 1 and Grade 3. Stage 1 meant it was small. Grade 3 meant it was a fast grower. I don't want to call it aggressive, but let's call a spade a spade here. With it being Grade 3 was in a way a good thing being as the cells were multiplying quickly, the chemo usually worked really well on this type of cancer.

After we found all this out, Dr. H walked us to the scheduler's desk. I am sure I looked like a deer in headlights to her as she hugged me and told me it will be ok. **It will be okay** she told me again as the hug go a little tighter. I wanted to hold on to those words for dear life. Eric and I were sitting at the chemo scheduler's desk and she asked, "So when do you want start?" This question took me a few minutes to wrap my head around. When do I want to start? Well hell, was there ever a good day to start chemo?

"Never" I said with a nervous laugh. Thinking to myself, I never want to start this shit. I ended up picking Friday. I don't know why I said Friday. I just kind of blurted it out. But after thinking about it more and talking to a few people I called and moved my chemo day to Monday. From what I heard through the grapevine, more than likely I will feel the worst a few days after each treatment. I don't want to feel my worst every other weekend. I would rather feel the worst during the week, when Ian won't be home to see me feeling like crap and Eric will be at work with his mind off of this mess. Maybe? Hopefully?

Chemo will last 16 weeks. I will be on a bi-weekly cycle which is considered very aggressive, but they had found with triple negative, if a person can handle the aggressive schedule, the tumor responds much better. And with me being young and healthy, she feels the more aggressive schedule will work for me. I hope so, let's get this over with. The first 8 weeks I would be on Adriamycin and Cytoxan or A/C for short. The second 8 weeks I will be on Taxol. The A/C is supposed to be the worst of it. I will lose my hair somewhere within two to three weeks after starting. It can cause extreme fatigue, and a lot of other things that I didn't read. Who cared at this point? All I know was it all sounded like a load of shit and I didn't want any part of it. The Taxol isn't supposed to be as bad and my hair might even start growing back during this time. Yeah I guess?!

I do realize this is going to be a very trying four months. I just keep telling myself, it is just four months. Not all that long in the grand scheme of things. I also realize these four months will change me forever. I am just ready to get started so I can be done. And, we already have a cruise planned for February 14th and if all goes according to plan, we will be on the cruise ship celebrating my cancer free body.

Okay....bye?!??? – October 2, 2008

Leaving work on Friday was surreal. Knowing that I would not be returning for at least sixteen weeks and trying to get everything either taken care of or passed to someone else, made this all so real. It wasn't like when I was preparing to leave for maternity leave, which was such a happy time. I mean I was leaving to have a baby, to add a bundle of joy to our world. Leaving this time, I had to stand up straight and face the truth. I was going on leave to fight for my life. Saying good bye didn't come so easily this time around. None of us knew what was really going to happen. We all wanted to think we knew, but it showed on all of our faces. It showed that none of us really knew if they would see me again.

We were scared for me, scared of the unknown future.

Work for me had always been such a safe place. I knew what to expect there; although, some days were far from normal. But, I knew my job so well and those I worked with, I could walk through my days with confidence knowing I KNEW what was going on. Leaving that safe place made me feel so unsafe and so unconfident in what was about to happen in my life.

Mascara – October 3, 2008

Today was the first day since I heard the news that I had worn mascara. No, not because all my eyelashes have already fallen out. I wondered if they really will? Eh, whatever. I wore it again today and will continue to wear it daily because I decided there will be no more tears shed to this illness. I have realized that I have so much to be thankful for and I am so much to so many people, I didn't have time to cry about what might be – I only have time to be thankful for what is.

I started thinking about how many people are in my life and how many people are already praying for me, and how many people need me and I am truly overwhelmed with the pure love I felt just thinking about it. So with that in mind, I made a list of who I was and need/want to be for the people in my life and who I love to be for them.

I Am...

A mother to Ian – he needs me. He needs me to be his mom, to hold him when he is hurt, to help him get over his first heart ache, to help him understand the world – he needs me. Plain and simple, he needs his mom.

A wife to Eric – he needs me to keep him company, hold hands with and just love him. He needs me to tell him all my crazy ideas and him be able to help me figure out a way we can make them a reality.

A sister – Rachele needs me more than she will ever admit. She is the older of us two, but she needs me to help her believe there is still magic in the world. She looks at the world as most analytical people do – black or white. But she needs me to help her see all the crazy colors swirled around. She needs me to be her little sister who she can help me find my way when I am lost.

A daughter to my mom and dad – they both need me in such different ways. My mom needs me to talk to. She needs me to be her little girl still to protect from the big bad world. She needs me to need her. Dad needs me to talk to him and let him know how much he means to me. He needs me to call him and just talk. He needs me like Rachele needs me too – to have my crazy dreams that I go after. Sometimes I fall and they are there to pick me up, but sometimes I fly and they are there to cheer me on.

A daughter-in-law and sister-in-law – they need to know Eric is so loved and is happy. They need to know that Eric is taken care of and they don't need to worry about his happiness.

A friend – they all need me to be there for them. To listen to them, give advice to them although it is sometimes unsolicited advice, to laugh with them, to make them laugh, hug and be hugged, and this is just the tip of it all. We all need each other in this life.

An aunt - to wonderful kids that need a fun and "hip" aunt. I want to be that aunt they know they can talk to when they don't want to talk to their own parents. That aunt they know they can count on.

A granddaughter, a niece, a cousin and much more to so many. I am so much to so many others and when I think of this, all I can think of is, how blessed am I to have all these people in my life who need ME? And I need them. So with that, I don't have time to feel sorry for myself. All I have time for is to enjoy everyone around me. And help them see their beauty as well. Please, if you take anything away from me sharing my story with you as I am going through this, take away this. Look at those in your life and know how blessed you are for what you have. And don't be afraid to tell them you love them.

Bubbly and cheese – October 4, 2008

Eric and I are drained, both physically and emotionally. We have been trying to carry on as normal, as if we didn't have this huge gray cloud hanging over our heads threatening to send a bolt of lightning down at any minute. It is exhausting. But I pushed all that aside and decided I wanted to feast the weekend before everything started and really have one more "normal" weekend. Whatever normal actually is anymore? We put Ian to bed and popped a bottle of bubbly for me and Eric. We both needed something of our old life to really cling to and an at-home date night is it. Crackers and cheese was on the menu for dinner. Oh yes, we are that fancy! Candles filled the darkness with just enough light, and Nora Jones played on the CD player.

For a moment in time, I was able to forget what was just ahead of me. It seemed our problems all just melted away like the wax on the candle that was burning in front of us.

We started doing living room picnics after Ian was born and we were no longer able to just go on a whim. Oh, how Ian has changed us in so many ways. We ate cheese, drank champagne, held each other and tried not to cry. We tried our best not to cry, but it didn't work for long. We cried in each other's arms and we cried some more.

The Day before it all begins…a happy jumbled mess – October 5, 2008

I didn't know quite how to feel today. I cried on and off all day. It would sneak up on me and take my surprise every time. I mean, I am starting chemo tomorrow. What will that really bring? There is no manual for this. People can tell you their experience, but what does that mean for me? If I am honest with myself right at this moment I feel like a tornado is ripping me apart piece by piece, and laughing in my face just because it can.

I feel sad.

I feel sad for me, for Eric, for Ian.

I feel excited in some weird way. Not to start chemo, but to know I am actively doing something about this crap.

I feel scared. Scared like the night before I went in to be induced for labor with Ian. I had no idea what I was actually in for. After 14 long hard hours, I ended up having to have a C-section. He was side-ways and I couldn't take the pain of them flipping him again. Yes it was attempted many times.

Church was hard today. I cried like a baby. I stood there and wept all service long. I am still not sure what stirred inside of me to make me cry like I did, but I just felt so moved there and so connected to my spirit and God, I was brought to tears. This was a very humbling experience for me to show my emotions so openly to a room full of strangers. Those emotions are usually reserved for my family and my close friends. Very few people in my life have ever seen my cry before and I realized today that was because I never wanted to make myself vulnerable to anyone. It was actually a very liberating experience to cry without inhibitions and not care what anyone thought about it.

People called all day to wish me luck tomorrow. We all tried to talk around the real reason they were calling, but it hung thick in the air no matter what way we all tried to steer the conversation. All the calls all ended up the same, everyone in tears, love being sent over the phone lines and virtual hugs. We all prayed together. We all gathered all the courage we could find. Eric and I talked more, cried more, hugged more, and then we both said it was time. It was time to stand up straight, put our body armor on and go into battle – hand in hand.

Chemo Chronicle #1 – October 6, 2008

I was actually able to sleep last night which really surprised me because usually when I am anxious, I don't sleep well. That wasn't the case. I dreamt that it was 8:15 and my mom was still blow drying her hair. I was so upset that she was going to make me late for my first day of chemo. Needless to say, that was not the case and Eric and I were right on time at 8:20. I didn't put my numbing cream on early enough so I did feel them stick me in the chest. Nothing like a needle in the chest to wake you up for the day! They were able to draw blood through the port also, so no need to get any additional sticks today. Yeah for only one stick!! It is funny the things I think are on the bright side now.

I was back in the "chemo room" around 9:30.This was such a crazy place. I felt 100% like Alice in Wonderland with all these different characters around and never knowing what to expect around the next corner. It looked like a sea of metal poles with IV bags hanging down. I wondered if they were all on the same chemo as me, surely not. Beeps were going off all over the room. I never knew where they were coming from or when the next one would blare out. It never failed, I got startled every time one blew its horn. I didn't even know why they were beeping. There were 6 rows of 5 reclining chairs, so all in all over 30 chairs for people to sit and receive some kind of life-saving drug. It held a whole new perspective when I looked at it that way. All kinds of people were there - some with hair, some without, some so skinny they looked like they could blow away if there was a gust of wind, some men, some women, some sleeping, some watching TV, some here with someone, some here by themselves. No one was the same as his or her neighbor. It was like a community in there, just a little bit of everyone. I had several neighbors around me. We were all lying in the chairs that reclined and the chairs looked comfortable until I was actually laying in it. Some of us had company with us and some did not. My heart was sad for those who were there by themselves.

I guess it is true when they say cancer doesn't discriminate. There truly was all walks of life in here. After all that eyeing of the other clientele, it was my turn to start. I felt like I was being asked to walk a tight rope over an alligator pit. One misstep and who knows what might happen? My nurse came over to read me the all too thick stack of paper telling me all the possible side effects of all these liquids that were about to be dripped into my body, telling me if I felt like I couldn't breathe to let him know, and good luck because the ride was starting. I signed all these papers saying that I understood all the risks. I found it highly ironic that these drugs which were going to kill the cancer to save my life could kill me too. I didn't tell my nurse that though. I thought it was much too early in the game for me to be a complete smart ass. And whatever, I didn't really even read all those papers that I signed. I didn't want to. It didn't matter one way or another to me. I still had to get the chemo no matter what those papers said. Eric read through them with a fine tooth comb and that was fine with me. At least one of us would know if something totally crazy happens it could be a reaction to the chemo. They wheeled over my pole that held the IV bags up high. Higher than me standing up which is 5 foot 10 inches. My first hook up of the day was to saline which just made me cold. I was so glad someone had told me to bring a warm, cozy blanket. All these liquids that were being pumped into me are at room temp, so they make me cold. And the room was cold because the nurses were hot from running around so much. I guess cancer is a cold bitch all around!! If you didn't know better, it kind of looked like a game of freeze tag going on. You had to stop moving when your nurse got to you to do what needed to be done. Next up, a tiny bag of steroids and another bigger bag of major anti-nauseous medicine, these two ran together. I started out watching the drips from the bag go down the tubes to the IV which eventually ended up in my port and then my body. After 5 minutes of that I decided I couldn't do that for the whole 4-5 hours. Seriously, I might go mad if I sat and watched this all day. Here we go - I received my first bag of chemo at 10:10. This was the C of the A/C. While lying there receiving this medicine, my sinuses started hurting. Like when you breathe in cold-dry-mountain air that makes your face feel like it might shattered from the cold. Then my nose started itching like crazy. None of the reading material warned me of this. The Cytoxan was pumped in for an hour and then the A of the A/C had to be manually pushed in for 15 minutes. They call the A, the red devil because it is literally red and can cause some nasty side effects. Nice, just what I want in my body. It was odd though. When I got up to leave, I asked my nurse if I was supposed to feel bad now or what?! I mean, I just got 2 bags of chemo pumped into me, and I was leaving there feeling fine. He told me to wait about 24 hours and I should start experiencing my fun! One down and only seven to go.

The Next Day – October 7, 2008

Ian woke up around 5:30 a.m., so I went in and rocked him back down to sleep. The way I looked at it was if I felt good enough to rock him, I wanted to. All my problems seemed to float away as I glided him to sleep. I had to go get a shot of Neulasta at 1:15. I would have to get this shot the day after every chemo infusion to boost my white blood cell count. It may or may not cause bone pain. I love all the maybes I get to deal with here.

Waiting for the train – October 8, 2008

I felt like I was sitting here waiting for the train to hit me, but I so badly didn't want to think that way. I was still holding on to my hope that I was not going to be affected as badly by chemo as some people were. But come on let's call a spade a spade. I did realize I was going to have some side effects. I just had poison dripped into my body. But when were they going to come and what would they be? I was still really tired but I think a lot of that was due to me not sleeping well at night. The steroids they gave me at treatment made me hyper and then the anti-nausea medicine I took were supposed to make me sleep, but it didn't work last night. They told me I could take Tylenol PM as well, so I am going to get some of that today and hopefully sleep tonight.

Pregnant?? – October 10, 2008

No I am not, but man I feel like it. This is the best way I can describe how I feel and most women who have been pregnant might be able to relate. I am about 50% more tired than I was my first trimester of pregnancy. I seem to have this cloud over my head constantly zapping energy. I am not doing more than I was, actually less but I am exhausted, all day, and all the time. And I am only on #1 treatment of my 8.

Food - Friend or foe? Just like with my first trimester, the only things that sound good was junk food. Think tater tots, chilly dogs, etc...

Sad with regret – October 13, 2008

Today while I was sitting at the oncologist waiting to be called back for my blood work I glanced over and observed a young women breast feeding her daughter in the waiting area. It was a bitter sweet moment for me. I loved seeing this mother care for her child like this, but it also made me so sad, so sad for so many reasons, sad with regret. Breast feeding didn't go as I had planned with Ian. It was hard, and I wonder if I gave up too easily. I was able to give him breast milk for 4 months but it took a lot of work. It was a daily challenge for me. And at the time, it was just easier for me to pump and let Eric help with the night feedings. I had always said, with number two, I would try harder and not give up as easily.

But it hit me today, what if I didn't get a second chance? What if I didn't get to make right all these decisions I made then? What if I didn't get a number two? My heart broke as I sat there and mourned for the loss of what might never be. But, that was a reminder for me today, tomorrow and all the days after, never say, I will do it next time. I have to do it this time because I might not have a next time.

A Fine line - October 14, 2008

I have noticed I walk a fine line, a very fine line between feeling great and doing too much and being exhausted. I felt fantastic this morning and went over to help a friend make birth announcements, and to hold her sweet little babies. I got home around 3:00 and totally crashed. It was so aggravating to me to feel so good but not be able to do what I normally did. I know I am on chemo treatment, but I don't feel "sick". It is really hard for me to wrap my head around me being this tired. There are so many things I want to do, but I literally can't or I will crash and burn.

So here I am, like a zombie robot. My body hurt from being tired. I am trying not to beat myself up for being so tired when my boys got home, for me not unloading the dishwasher, for the pile of laundry sitting on the couch and all the other things I thought I should be doing. All at the same time, I am trying to understand this invisible line that seems to move up and down all the time.

That line. Oh that line.

That line that when I do cross over it, all the plates that I have piled up topple over and crash to the ground. I will inevitably cross this line again during this whole treatment process because I am stubborn. I don't learn things the first time around. And I think I can do the same thing and somehow change the outcome. I need to understand the outcome will be the same if I push too hard.

I have been warned that I will more than likely be even more tired with less of an appetite than I was from the first treatment, but if that is the worst of it, I can and will take it. My blood counts all look good still and the best news of all, Dr. H says the tumor feels smaller and not as dense. Eric had said the same thing, but it just holds so much more merit hearing it from her. I left there feeling tired and with a side of nausea.

So it begins…- October 21, 2008

I think. Well I know. I am about to start losing my hair. I was just giving Ian kisses and he pulled a ton of hair out. It didn't even hurt so you can image my surprise after I was done kissing him to look at him holding two handfuls of hair. At first I thought, what in the hell is that? Only to quickly remember that it was about time for my hair to start falling out.

Bad Day – October 22, 2008

Today has hands down been the worst day yet. My tummy was giving me problems again and my hair was really starting to fall out all over the place. I woke up to piles of hair on my pillow and face. After dreaming I had a feather boa on that was choking me.

While in the shower washing my hair, I could just pull out handfuls. Every time I touched my hair more hail came out.

I broke.

I really broke down.

I don't know how long I stayed in the shower crying. After I got out, I was wiped out, so I went back to bed. I did decide though that in order to keep semi control of this situation, I was going to do something about it. I was going to have Eric shave my head.

Butterfly – October 27, 2008

At 4:00 yesterday afternoon I was tired of my hair hurting, my head itching and feeling like I was sheading everywhere. I was very ready to have Eric shave it off.

I decided we should make it a party seeing as how I never planned on doing this again. So many people showed up to help show Eric and I much love. Everyone brought food and drinks and we all forgot for a few minutes the reason we were all here.

Then it was time. If this was going to happen, we needed to get this show on the road.

The actual process of having it shaved felt odd being as I have never had my head shaved before. The buzz of the razor on my head was definitely a first. Watching the clumps of hair fall to the ground was a hard for me. It made it all so real again and again. After every clump feel to the ground, it sunk in a little more. It took me a minute to look at myself in the mirror after I had an official buzz cut. I didn't know what to expect. Was it still going to be me?

Eric brought me out a mirror. I looked and I must say I was pleasantly surprised. I have had many hair styles and/or colors over the course of my life. In the past after I drastically change my hair, every time I would walk by a mirror I would have to do a double take to make sure that was still me. I was expecting this to be the same but for some reason, it wasn't. This felt natural and was freeing in a way I never knew was possible. While I was looking at my hair on the ground and taking everything in, a butterfly appeared out of nowhere. I am not sure who all saw it, but Eric and I saw it at the same time. I felt like it was here to let us both know that things were going to be okay. I was in my cocoon struggling to get out at the moment but it wouldn't be long until I was ready to fly and spread beauty throughout the world.

Inspiration – November 6, 2008

I heard the other day that we should try to find inspiration in our day to day lives everywhere we look. We watched "Dan in Real Life" the other night and I found a great deal of inspiration in a quote from the movie. "The only thing you can plan on in life is to plan to be surprised." Now, it took a while for this to really set in with me and then it hit me. I realized how much my timeline in life is now a surprise to me and out of my hands.

While rocking Ian to sleep last night, after a few sips of water he didn't want to be rocked to sleep. He wanted to be put in bed and fall asleep on his own. It made me realize how sad it made me for my timeline; my timeline that I had been imaging in my mind for so long now. If my body was mine right now, we would be trying to get pregnant again. I want another baby so badly. But this has made me realize no matter what we plan, how well that plan is laid out in our heads and hearts, it doesn't matter. It isn't up to us. I truly believe God has a plan laid out for each and every one of us. Sometimes it takes a little kick in the pants to get us to realize that plan. Now, I am not entirely sure what the plan is for me and my family but I do know that whatever happens, I will now always plan to be surprised.

Great Expectations – November 9, 2008

I have always tried not to expect anything from any given situation or anyone because in my mind, if I don't expect it, I can't be let down. Now don't get me wrong, I HOPE for the best in every situation and from every person. I just don't expect it from any one thing or anyone.

Sometime during my first two treatments, I started to expect that I would bounce back by the weekend following a treatment and I could breeze through the rest of my treatments as easily as I had the first two.

Since I was expecting to feel better by the weekend and it was now the weekend, I was now let down that I was still completely exhausted and my body hurt because I was so tired. I can't fight this feeling of disappointment in myself. On a logical level I knew this wasn't my fault. But truth be told, I was disappointed that I ever let myself believe this was going to be a breeze. It isn't easy. I was tired all the time but I just kept telling myself, I could be SO much worse. I mean, honestly, yes I was exhausted and had a funky burnt taste in my mouth but there were so many other side effects I could be experiencing and was not and for that I was truly blessed and grateful for. So, I don't want to come across as ungrateful for how well I am doing here because I am but I am getting tired of being tired.

And all I could really think of right now was I only had one more A/C treatment and then I was halfway done with my 8 chemo treatments. But then reality kicked in, I was still not even halfway done and I was sick of this shit. I wanted my life back. I wanted my body to be mine again and not under attack from cancer and a counter attack of a violent chemical.

Chemo Chronicle #5 – December 1, 2008

Today's chemo session was hands down the worst, hardest and longest session yet. We got to the office at 8:30, and I talked to my doctor and all was well there. I was hooked up to a huge bag of Benadryl at 9:00. I was hoping that was going to knock me out but it didn't. It was just enough to put me over the edge into la-la land. I couldn't even do anything to pass the time because nothing made sense to me. I was given the Benadryl because the Taxol can cause major allergic reactions in some people. One of the first signs of a reaction is a dry cough. I already had a cough before chemo started. It was winter, and I had a kid in daycare. Enough said. All the nurses were on high alert with me all day because of my cough, which in turn made me very anxious and stressed out. I would try to hold in my coughs then that would make it all the worse. The few times I had to use the restroom, Eric had to stand outside the door because I couldn't lock the door in case I had a reaction. Unfortunately, I knew these reactions they were telling me about were in fact real because a lady on the next row had a reaction to the treatment she was on. All the doctors came running and nurses swarmed. It was crazy and so scary. But now I knew why they were taking my cough so seriously.

So, there I was thinking at any minute I could have a reaction all the while putting my hands and feet in ice baths. Why on earth was I putting my hands and feet in freezing water in the middle of December one might wonder? One of the side effects of Taxol can be nerve damage to the hands and feet. If I were to get said nerve damage, it would make my hands and feet feel like they were asleep all the time. And from what I have heard, it can be extremely painful. Honestly it wasn't the pain part that scared me. The thought of me not being able to use my hands to create things is what scared me more. That is why I decided to do the ice bath and I will continue to do them the next three times as well. I can't say keeping my hands and feet in ice water was easy. It sucked big time. Then I started feeling sick to my stomach, which I think was from not eating so Eric went and got us sandwiches. That started to help but didn't totally take it away. After eating and while doing the ice bath, I started having hot flashes also. Nice. How was I having hot flashes while having my hands and feet in ice I will never know? I was miserable. My cough was getting much worse at this point and everyone was freaking out. My nurse suggested cough medicine which I had a prescription for the whole time but none of us thought to get it filled there at that pharmacy.

This was when I broke. I just started crying. I didn't feel good from my cold and not to mention having chemo dripped into me. My cough was driving me nuts and had everyone on edge. I just wanted to go home.

While Eric was at the pharmacy getting the medicine, the lady next to told me what a wonderful husband I had. And when Eric was making my appointment for the surgery consult, my nurse was telling me how lucky I was to have Eric there with me every time and the support he gives me isn't what he sees every day. I know all this and will be eternally grateful for him in my life. He also told me I couldn't ever cry like that in front of him again because it broke his heart. He is truly a caring nurse.

My stomach was still on edge, so they ordered a bag full of medicine that in pill form made me pass out. I was truly expecting to go limp in the chair and completely pass out. I didn't. I just couldn't let go of my anxiety enough to let myself drift off. When it was all finally over, I had to hold on to Eric's arm in order to actually walk out though. Too bad I don't have a good party story to go along with this day like I would back in day when Eric would have to come pick me and my friend, Laurie, up from happy hour. Oh times have changed – times have changed. I miss my other life. That was one of the longest days ever but it is over now. We came home and I was finally able to pass out for a few hours and woke up to something great – our Christmas tree was up!! I kept reminding myself that no matter how bad this day was, it is over now and I only have 3 more treatments left!

Different.... December 3, 2008

All I can say about this treatment is that the effects have been much different from A/C. I am not sure they are worse or how to describe them, but I do have the bone pain they warned me about. The best way I can describe it is it feels like "growing pains" we all experienced when getting a growth spurt. I have these bone pains mainly in my lower back, calf bones and ankles. My doctor told me I could take pain medicine for them. I really don't want to be looped out all day, so I am going to try to get through them.

Prayers – December 4, 2008

I am not sure if I have ever openly solicited prayers for myself from others, but I am doing it now. I am trying really trying not to let this one horrible day break me.

It can't break me.

It won't break me.

I am afraid I wouldn't be able to be put back together.

I want to enjoy the holidays like I used be able to and not deal with any of this right now.

From my waist down, my bones hurt so badly. I can barely stand or walk because of the pain that radiates through my body. The bottom of my feet feel like they are on fire when I stand on them, so to say the least I have been laying on the couch all day; which really isn't comfortable either because my hips hurt too. So yes, I am asking for prayers for myself, for this bone pain to go away and for strength to make it through the remaining three chemos.

Minor breakdown – December 5, 2008

Yes, yesterday was awful but I think in some weird way it helped me to cry and let it all out. I wanted to be strong all the time but it was hard to hold onto that I'm okay face all the time. Yesterday, I just couldn't do it anymore. I let it all go. I let all the pain, fear, anger, sadness go. I let it all go. I couldn't carry the load anymore. After allowing others to help me up and walk away, I was leaving my own pity party. I had to get my mind back in this game. This was almost over. I only had 3 more treatments left. I was 62.5% done with chemo treatments. I would do whatever it took. I would get myself through this.

Chemo Chronicle #6 – December 15, 2008

I really didn't want to go to chemo today. I wondered what they would do if I just didn't show up? Would it be like skipping school? Would they call Eric and ask where the hell I am? This had been the only Monday thus far that I really hadn't wanted to go. I was trying and trying hard to pray that it wasn't as bad as last time. The chemo room was hopping today and a little backed up. I saw my doctor promptly at 9:00 for about 15 minutes. But I didn't get hooked up until 10:00 and we left at 2:30.

I made a few friends while Eric was out getting us lunch. It worked out much better this time because I ate right when I started getting hungry versus waiting until I was starving. I really think this helped me not get so nauseous. I tweaked the ice bath process too. Instead of putting my hands with latex gloves on directly in a bowl of ice, I brought freezer bags and held the bag of ice. For my feet, I had on thin socks and put bags over my feet while I put them in a tub of ice. My feet weren't bad at all because they numbed up quickly. I would like to say this is getting easier, but I would be lying.

Christmas Time – December 2008

Christmas came and went and I can't believe it.

I wish I could say it was be a holly jolly Christmas, but I just couldn't get my heart into it.

My mind was going crazy with wanting to get every little detail done and perfect, but I just didn't have it in me. I have did a lot of shopping on-line and honestly didn't buy stuff for a lot of people I usually do. I was tired and honestly, didn't care.

The colder it got the more my bones hurt. Nice huh? I was afraid I wasn't going be able to hold it together to make it through Christmas.

I was afraid that all the emotions in me that I kept stuffing down, were going to break the surface sooner rather than later. I never thought I would say all I wanted for Christmas was to not have cancer.

As usual, we went at my sister's house and Ian was in cousin heaven.

Too many gifts lined the floor and were stacked high. I hoped the stacks didn't topple over.

Mom and Rachele wrapped gifts with big, fun bows that made you not want to open them because they was too pretty.

Not me. Not this year at least. All my gifts were in gift sacks.

Family, church, too many cookies, yummy food, fun on the new trampoline, board games, and more family, and then it was over just like that. I didn't want to leave my sister's house. I felt that I could pretend my life was normal here. It was time though. We had to leave, so I could be back for chemo on Monday. Cancer doesn't take holidays off.

Chemo Chronicle #7... – December 29, 2008

And with the end of this one, I am walking on sunshine because I ONLY HAVE ONE LEFT!!! One chemo treatment left! Being as my blood work looked so good, I don't have to get a shot tomorrow! I am praying I will feel better all-around Wednesday, Thursday, Friday and Saturday since I don't have to get the shot. I am still expecting the flu like symptoms, but those won't be near as bad without the bone pain.

The chemo room was hopping today. My nurse said it was because people tried to get one more treatment in before the end of the year and new set of insurance deductibles. That made sense. This treatment wasn't too bad. I did the ice therapy again on my hands and feet. Again, my feet numbed up quick and didn't really bother me, my hands were a lot more difficult to keep in the ice for long periods of time, but I did it. All I kept thinking about was the gifts I wanted to make for a friend's baby shower, the cute Valentine gift ideas I had in mind and all the stuff I so enjoyed doing. In my mind, a few hours of pain in ice was so worth it to have all the feeling in my hands for my lifetime.

Eric got us sandwiches again for lunch which helped so much to eat there versus getting too hungry. I noticed a lot of younger woman such as myself today. A few I had seen before, but there were many I hadn't ever seen. I did wonder why they were there. Did they have cancer too? Oh, one lady got to ring the bell today. I will get to ring it next week. On your last chemo treatment day, you get to right the bell and they throw confetti at you. I am going to ring the hell out of that bell – hell yes I am!!

Love Actually… - December 31, 2008

Love actually **is** all around. I didn't come up with that line myself I just watched one of my favorite movies – Love Actually. And it is true, love actually is all around. I was at the post office yestered and a woman walked up to me, and asked if she could ask me a personal question. I smiled and said yes. She asked if I was going through chemo and when I said yes, she gave me a cute scarf she made. She told me a little of her story; when she was going through chemo, her sister made her lots of scarves. She wanted to pass on the love she felt from her sister to others. I was honored to receive it. She asked me where I was at in my treatment, asked me if I was able to eat and told me not to worry about all the little shit in life because it just isn't worth it. How awesome was that for a total stranger to share so much of herself with me because she noticed I didn't have hair? She took it upon herself to take a chance and come ask me something very personal.

Opening up is scary stuff. I think it is most scary to open up to myself, then to share it with others. Once I say it out loud it is real. Every thought has meaning and emotion behind and it is nothing to be embarrassed about it. This is one of the life lessons I am not sure if I would have learned without cancer invading my life. You know what, this is just another reason I am thankful for cancer. Now don't get me wrong, I am ready for it to be gone forever, but I "ok" it was here for a bit.

2009

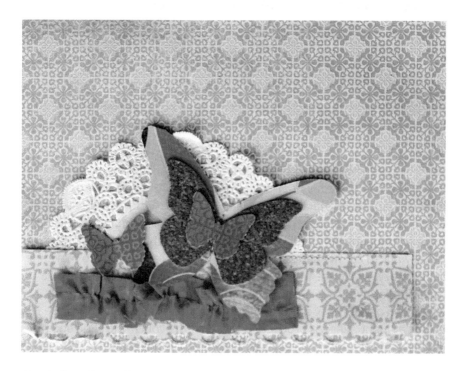

Anticipation - January 8, 2009

Really...how can my last chemo appointment be only 4 days away? It seemed like I just found the lump a few weeks ago.

I have an appointment with my breast surgeon on January 15th. I don't know what all this will involve but I have a questions concerning the lumpectomy.

Is it true I might not be able to raise my arm above my head?

Can I develop lymphoma (swelling of the arm)?

That was my next step though. I needed to finish this step first, I kept reminding myself. Once this step was done, and surgery was complete, then next step was to start thinking about radiation.

"They" say it is so much easier than chemo. Here's hoping whoever they are, are right.

Taxol hasn't been that bad. I have been having an odd issue though... itchy hands. This was the third time this has happened after Taxol, so I knew it was due to Taxol.

These itch attacks suck big time. Here was how the itch breaks down. It slowly starts Thursday or Friday after chemo with just a little itch here or there on my hands, fingers and wrists. Saturday it starts to get worse and I have to scratch my hands on my jeans. Sunday, I feel like I am scratching my hands all day on anything I can. By Monday, I pretty much want to cut my hands off because the itch really starts to make me a little crazy. Of course there are medications for this itch, as there is a medicine for everything. But, this medicine made me drunk. Literally, I was drunk about thirty minutes after I took this stuff. I try not to take it except at night, where I proceeded to lay on the couch with Eric and he laughs at me because I guess I say some pretty funny stuff...

Here we go again... - January 16, 2009

I get to start all the tests again to see if I am really clean and clear. Yesterday, I had a PEM scan to check that no cancer is hiding in the ole boobs. I forgot how bad those suck. Nothing like having each boob smashed 3 different ways for 10 minutes at a time. This is NO exaggeration!

But honestly, I really thought I was done with all these tests.

I don't know why I thought this.

I guess I need to get used to getting scanned on a regular basis. From the sound of what Dr. H told me, I will be getting some sort of scan every 6 months for quite some time.

The surgeon visit was kind of pointless yesterday, except for the fact that when she felt for the cancer, she said she couldn't even find it!! Good news there.

Other than that, she told me about the tests I will need before we do surgery. The lymph node removal still seems to be the most difficult part of the surgery. I guess I will see.

Speechless –January 26, 2009

The results from my scan came in and drum roll please...there were no notable areas of concern in either breast! That means, if it would have looked like this in the beginning, they wouldn't have recognized it as cancer. Oh happy days!! The chemo sucked but it worked, IT WORKED!! I asked if I still had to have surgery. And yes, yes I did but I didn't even care about that! All I cared about was that the cancer was dead.

One More Chapter... - February 1, 2009

And just like that, one more chapter of this journey has come to an end! I am one step closer to being done with cancer and getting back to my normal life. The results of all the pathology is in and I am FREE AND CLEAR! Nothing was found in the lymph nodes and the margins of cancer were clear. Dr. H. said this was the best possible outcome we could have hoped for. HELL YES it was! I am really thankful this chapter is coming to a close and so ready to move on from it. It has consumed my life for the past 4 months and I am over it. I don't want to forget it though; I have to remind myself of what I have gotten through and how I have grown from it. And as odd as this sounds, it is kind of a hard for me right now. Before this whole cancer bit happened, my normal life revolved around family, friends, work, etc. Then life shifted to figuring out what was going on with me. The testing, the waiting, and the decisions of everything that was being thrown at us and that consumed us for a month. That month seemed like forever. Then we were told it was cancer and I had that to deal with that; had to wrap my mind around dealing with how to handle the cancer part of this and the side effects of the treatments. All the while, I was trying to hold it all together for myself and more so for Eric and Ian. Now in a blink of my eyes, it is gone. I am now called a cancer survivor. But now what? My life was flipped upside down and now it was being handed back to me but I had to ask, do I want it back the way it was? I don't think so. I don't want to live blindly and take simple things for granted, like holding Ian. Before any of this happened, I would think my goodness Ian is so heavy, or not exercising when I was perfectly capable of exercising...I just didn't feel like it because I was being lazy. Or not telling people in my life why I love them or why they are special to me. I don't want to go back to that person. But how do I remember that without rehashing the hard times of chemo, which I don't want to do.

How do I come into this new life? It is scary for me in so many ways and empowering at the same time.

One month later – February 13, 2009

It has been one month since my last chemo. I continue to feel a little better every day, but then I do too much and crash again. My skin is flaking off and I have a few mouth sores, which suck big time. I assume this was happening because the dead skin was coming off but I don't know for sure. I do know it isn't fun. Even my lips are peeling. Really, my lips, oh yes! Oh, and my eyebrows and eye lashes are falling out now. My doctor did say this was because they are slow growing hair follicles, so it takes longer for them to fall out. Nice. I am not too concerned about the eye lashes, it is the eyebrows that I don't want to go. I thought maybe I should start penciling them in with funny expressions? Or not?

After seeing my oncologist last week, I realizing more of the impact of me being 100% pathologically recovered. She said it was something for me to be very grateful for being as only 20% of people respond that well to chemo. She gave me an A+! I will go see my radiation doctor on February 24th. I am not sure if I will start radiation that day or soon after. Honestly, I hope I start that day to get my 6 weeks rolling and finished.

I have to get radiation still to "mop the floor" of any possible lingering cells. No I don't want to get radiation for 6 weeks, but I would so much rather do this now then have to go through all the other stuff I went through again.

Telling the truth – March 3, 2009

Why is telling the truth about something that you don't want to face so hard to do?

I guess I just answered my own question. In a way, once you say it out loud to others you aren't only telling your secret, you are also allowing yourself to know it is your truth.

I have had a rough couple of weeks and I couldn't quite put my finger on what was wrong. I had no motivation to do anything and when I say anything, I mean anything. Even on the cruise we just got back from, I wasn't me. I really didn't have fun because I was just blah. Everything completely stressed me out and I felt like I was "toeing the line" between ok and total meltdown every second of everyday.

When we got back, I didn't really want to be back, but I didn't want to be on the cruise either.

I didn't want to be creative.

I didn't want to talk to friends.

I didn't want to do anything that in my day to day life makes me happy.

I hit my breaking point last week when my radiation doctor told me that I will need radiation sessions – 35 of them.

Seven weeks…seven weeks total weeks of radiation.

I couldn't wrap my mind around 35 sessions nor could I pull myself out of the funk anymore.

I felt defeated, scared and tired of all this shit.

I called Dr. H and she told me post chemo depression was very common and actually didn't sound surprised by the fact I was calling.

Whatever, I was surprised.

No one ever talked to me about this beforehand.

I thought I had everything held together and packaged with a pretty bow in place for all to see...to see I was ok.

To see I beat cancer and didn't flinch.

Though, looking back, it was all held together with very fragile glue or wasn't held together at all.

I was put on anti-depressants and am praying they work and work fast. I know the feeling of depression all too well being as this isn't my first run in with the 3 headed monster I call depression.

A few day into me taking my "happy pill," I am starting to feel a lot better than I have felt in a long time.

So in my mind, they are already working. Maybe that was all I needed was the thought of getting better?

It is hard to explain to myself how I could let myself be depressed at this juncture of the journey. I have so much to be grateful for, I AM CANCER FREE, damn it. But I still have a lot of turmoil in me that I need to deal with and work out.

I think the reality of the situation in just now hitting me, the magnitude of what I went through is now in my face versus when I was going through it - I couldn't let it be in my face then.

If I let it get to me while I was going through it, I would have been defeated and THAT was not an option. So, it got to me a little later. Thankfully, I am stronger now and not afraid to tell the truth to myself and realize something was wrong.

I start radiation tomorrow and am scared. Scared of how it will actually be. It sounds painful in a completely different way than chemo was painful and different from how surgery was painful.

One - it is every flippin' freakin' day - Monday – Friday for seven weeks straight.

Two - what it will do to my skin sounds really painful. As in, I won't be able to wear a bra because it will hurt.

Three - fatigue is more than likely going to return.

I don't want to go, but I know I must. I try not to think about it too much. Again, there I go pushing stuff away. I try to remind myself that I have done so much these past five months and I will continue to do what I need to do to get through this and be done with it.

All I can picture is once I am done with radiation they will stamp my chart with a big, red CANCER FREE stamp on the outside of it. I am sure they don't actually do that but it sure would be nice if they did.

It is back – March 26, 2009

I am a little over 3 weeks into radiation and the side effects are starting in.

I am exhausted...exhausted all the time.

The extreme tiredness is really taking a toll on me.

The past few days I have had to take naps because my eyes just won't stay open. And these haven't been small naps; I sleep for a good 2 hours. I am not sure if it is because I have started going to bed a little later. A whopping 10:00pm. I feel like I could sleep all day but then I question myself and wonder if my happy pills aren't working the way they should or what in the hell is going on? I thought radiation was supposed to be easier!?!?!

So yes, I am a little down right now, just thinking about being tired makes me even more tired. I am going over to a friend's house after radiation to visit. I am really looking forward to that - Just getting out of my normal routine is a great change. And I am sorry for all these complaints - I feel like all I do is complain and honestly, I don't like it.

Bottle it up – March 27, 2009

I wish I could bottle up my happiness that I am experiencing today. I am not sure what happened between yesterday and today but something big did. I am honestly putting my money on answered prayers.

I have been so productive today, it is amazing me. I crafted and made "just because" cards. And it was kind of magical. I almost don't remember doing it. I was just in that place where things happen so easily and gracefully. When I noticed the happiness and ease I was feeling, I told myself to remember the feeling. When I am down to bring it out and remind me that yes, it is all going to be okay and I will get back to me someday soon.

SO close… - April 14, 2009

I am so close, but still so far away. The reality of my situation kind of smacked me in my face this morning. I really over did it this past weekend and have been paying for it the past two days. Paying for it as in needing 4 hour naps during the day and laying around the rest of time accomplishing nada. I still get so frustrated with myself when I do this. I push too hard to get too much done and then can't do anything because I have no energy.

And I got bad news today. My radiation doctor said we might have to hold off on radiation for a few days because my skin is really, REALLY burnt and it flippin' hurts and itches. He gave me a compress to use a few times a day followed by cream. The whole process takes around an hour of me needing to be topless and letting everything air dry. I have to continue this regimen 2-3 times a day until radiation is done. I will know tomorrow if I have to take a break or if can continue and hopefully finish next Wednesday! To say the least, I am so tired of all this crap. I am counting the days until I am done, whenever that is going to be.

My heart's song – April 16, 2009

I have tried to put this into words for a long time, but I just couldn't make it make sense. I feel I have to try again because something is telling me this is so very important. I watched an Oprah episode the other day and she talked about finding your heart's song. What is it that makes your heart sing? What makes your world go around? When money is set aside, what would you choose to do with your life? How would you help others? How would you make this world a better place to live? It is a hard question to answer because it is scary to take money out of the equation, but one huge thing I have realized through this journey, money does not and cannot make me happy. Yes, it makes life easier, but easy and happy are two totally different things.

I did something yesterday that I believe is taking me one step closer to my heart's song. I told my boss that I wouldn't be returning to work after I am done with all the treatments. After a lot of praying and many talks with Eric, I decided my heart wasn't/wouldn't be in it. I have to be true to my heart. Now, what is my heart's song? I am not 100% sure but I think I am getting closer to figuring it out. I know a huge piece of it is Ian. I don't know if we will get another baby, and I look at Ian and realize how fast time really goes. He is almost 2 years old and these first 2 years have flown by. I want to take every moment and be able to bottle it up as a memory. I want to leave my footprint on the world. I want to help people show their love to and for others. I want to show my love to and for others and so much more. I have a lot I want to do. Now, I just need to figure out how to start.

A switch - May 1, 2009

I got to walk through one more confetti shower today to celebrate my last radiation! It was a great feeling to know that I am done, really done. I would like to say to whoever told me radiation was easy I seriously want to punch them in the face. This was so far from easy as having my epidural wear off during my 14 hour labor. NOT.EASY.AT.ALL!! Of course it was doable, it is all doable. But the lack of energy, the pain in my boob all the time and the general idea of me being totally over this BS really hit me hard.

I am ready to jump into my next project. I was not sure what that will be, but I have a few ideas. I want to do something with my art to help others, but I'm just not sure how to go about it yet.

It is the small things – May 2, 2009

It truly is the small things in life that really make me happy these days. With me now out of work, I am learning again what to do that makes me happy that has nothing to do with money. My birthday is coming up, and I have had several people ask me what I want for my birthday. I can't think of one tangible item to tell them. If you would have asked me this in any year past, I would have a list of stuff that I would tell you. But this year, honestly all I want is my period to return. I want my energy to be back where it was a year ago. I want Ian to be happy and healthy. I want Eric to know how much I love him. I want to start showing people in my life how important they are to me without me expecting anything in return. I want to start exercising again and feel that rush of accomplishment after a hard workout class.

But back to the small things – I had two major firsts yesterday that a year ago wouldn't have even thought twice about but yesterday they were huge for me. One, I got up around 7:20 am. I know this sounds late, but

I had been sleeping until 9:30 am or 10:00 am and I didn't take a nap! I did lie down and read for an hour and went to bed at 10:00 pm. Two, I was able to wear a bra yesterday! HIP HORRAY!!! It felt really good to not have the burnt flesh hurting me at even the tiniest move. I am almost done peeling and decided yesterday I was done enough to wear a bra. And with that, I am thinking in about a week I should be able to wear a sports bra again and then I will be able to start working out. I guess my birthday wishes are all coming true even before my birthday!

Birthday – May 13, 2009

By definition a birthday is: 1) the anniversary of a birth 2) a day marking the beginning of something. I decided a few weeks ago that my birthday this year was going to be my "re-birth" and the beginning of something grand and magical. Thirty was a tough year for me and it was nothing as I expected it to be. I honestly thought I would be pregnant again sometime in my 30th year. I thought Eric and I would be looking at new houses for our expanding family. I thought I would be in the best shape of my life. (I am not sure why I thought this being as I hadn't even started working out or eating right.)

I thought a lot of things that just weren't meant to be. Instead of all those fabulous dreams, I got cancer. I am trying to learn from all this that I have gone through. I have learned, but I must say it is easy to forget how hard it was once it starts getting easy again. So with this new year, I am trying to muster up all my courage to embark on a journey. I am ready to take the path less taken and soar. Someone asked me the other night, would I rather have a seat belt or wings and without thinking I said wings. Then I asked her if that now means I am dead? No she gently said, that wasn't the point. Would you rather always be safe and secure and not be able to go anywhere or would you rather be able to fly – I would rather fly!

WHAT THE (*)#(*)CK??– May 15, 2009

I had a slight panic attack today at lunch. Ok, a full on panic attack. I went to a group lunch with a group of young breast cancer survivors. A new person joined so we went around and told our stories, and it came up that one lady was triple negative (same as me), went through chemo, lumpectomy and radiation (same as me) had a reoccurrence of cancer in the same spot. All that was running through my head was, What the F%#^K would I do with Ian if I got cancer again? Why didn't I just cut them off and call it good????

I left lunch in a panic, and called my support squad. Finally, Marci answered. I was ready to call Dr. H to schedule an appointment to take the girls off. But Marci reminded me of why I choose to keep the girls. I wanted to breast feed #2 and that was not an easy surgery contrary to what I had in my head about it. She reminded me that I was at peace with my decision. A decision Eric and I looked at every possible angle of before making. And that her story, it wasn't my story. I must admit, this was the first panic I had had since all this shit had started. Like Marci told me, I can't live my life by what ifs. I just can't. I guess what pisses me off about today the most is that I thought I was totally okay with everything. That I could go on my merry little way and the "cancer bit" was behind me and blah, blah, blah. But I am seeing that it is still a huge part of my life and more than likely will be forever and in a way it should be but I can't let it consume me. UGH!

Man alive…. – May 29, 2009

These past few days have almost done me in. I have had a lot going on and am kind of struggling to keep my head above water. I thought going through chemo, surgery, radiation was hard. I had no idea what was on the other side of the door for me! I am halfway kidding – halfway not. I am not going to lie this past week has been hard. I have wondered several times if I was physically and mentally ready for this? Am I really cut out to be a stay-at-home mom? Now stick with me here, I know I am capable of this new role in my life although it technically isn't new. I have been a mom since Ian was born, but the part of him depending on me for everything, and I mean **everything** scares me: kissing him when he is hurt, getting him breakfast, lunch, dinner and snacks, entertaining him all day long, and teaching him. I am so afraid I am not going to teach him what he needs to know and will somehow be behind when he goes to school. I don't know why I feel like this. I want everything for him in life and I don't want to be the reason he didn't/doesn't get to do something because I didn't teach him it. So with all this added stress in my life, the past two nights Eric has found me laid out on the couch after Ian is in bed eating chips and cookies.

Now, I know for him to say anything to me about what I was eating meant that he was really worried about me. He gently asked if I was okay because me laying there like that, eating that crap, was totally against all my new goals. When he first asked me about it, I was pissed off. How dare he ask me that when he had no idea what I felt like? After talking with him and realizing where he was coming from, I figured out I was totally comfort eating. I was freaking hungry all day, hungry like I was hungry when I was breast feeding. I didn't feel like I got a chance to eat because Ian wanted to eat what I was eating. I didn't eat junk in front of Ian because, well, I didn't want him eating it.

I am not sure where I am going with this, and I don't know how to sum it all and tie it together. Other than, I am tired, I am hungry, I have too much body fat on me but even after reading back through all this bitching and moaning, I can say I am happy. I love being able to kiss all of Ian's hurts away, watch him splash for hours in the pool, tell him to give people a beep and he does it and laughs and knowing he knows he can depend of me for all his needs and wants.

Life goes on – June, 2009

I had a follow appointment up with my radiation oncologist today with

Ian in tow and lesson learned; a toddler at a cancer building was good and bad. Good because all the patients were eating him up and bad because the employees looked at him for the germy little guy he is. My doctor was super impressed with where I was in regards to energy and what all I had been doing. He was even more impressed that I was at home all day with Ian and told me that if I have set backs in the weeks - even months to come to be easy on myself because he really had not seen anyone rebound back this quick after all I had been through. So, I guess with that, I will take his permission to slow down a bit and stop feeling guilty when I need to nap!

We drove to Florida for a vacation to see my best friend. It felt like life was returning to normal. I hate to use the word normal, but it is nice to be normal sometime. Ian started mother's day out two times a week because lets be totally honest here, I am not cut out to stay at home with him all day every day. I started working out again. I was very surprised how easy it was for me to start working out again and even more surprised at how much I missed the sweat sessions. I forgot how good my mind and body feel after a good sweat.

My Baby – August, 2009

My baby is turning 2 and in so many ways it is bitter sweet for me. I am so blessed to have such a happy, healthy, fun-loving little boy who loves his mommy and daddy so much but I am sad because I don't know what the future holds for us and more children. Two years old is SO different than one. He talks all the time, jumps from anything he can climb onto, tells me NO way too often and just loves life.

And his birthday party was a weird slap in the face. His birthday party last year was the last "normal" thing we did before I found the lump and life turned upside down. I guess I am just holding my breath to get through this birthday with no big surprises.

Me coming back – September, 2009

I guess you really never know how much you will miss somebody until that somebody is all the sudden not in your life anymore or how you wish you had become better friends with that somebody before they left. The saying is true, you don't know what you have until it is gone. Who I thought to be only an old acquaintance came back into my life this weekend and I realized this person was a long lost friend, someone whom without them with me left me with a void in my life for so many reasons, so many questions left unanswered, so many feelings left unsaid and a part of me was missing while she was gone. Who is the "someone" I speak so highly of?

Well, in reality it isn't an actual person at all, but a part of me. A part of all of us women, something we all take for granted, and something we all really love to hate. We all have a common bond to bitch about but without this something in your life, your womanhood is suddenly stripped from you and you are left wondering if you will ever be the same again? In so many ways that you never thought of before, because you had it and never remember life without it - our monthly cycle.MY PERIOD IS BACK! I cried like a baby Saturday morning when I realized what was happening. I cried for all I thought that was lost. I cried for me feeling whole again. I cried for this part of my journey finally coming to an end.

One year later – September 14, 2009

It has been once year since I heard the words that would ultimately change my life forever. "I am sorry, but it is cancer." I have been trying to wrap my mind around what I needed/wanted to write for this "anniversary" for about a week. It has been one year and 3 days since I heard those words. I never imagined I would be where I am at today a year ago when my world started spinning out of control. I reread all my old posts about the tests, the waiting, the scared nights of not sleeping; the fog that seemed to surround me, as the tears came flowing back so easily. I realized something that I had to have known then, but I couldn't say it out loud - I was scared to death. And I am trying not to let that fear come into my day-to-day life here and now.

I know we have all received an email, or 100 about "if we would have known then what we know now" and I now believe those have some validity. I have thought about it a lot and have thought about what I have learned from cancer and am very thankful for learning these lessons when I was 30 versus 90. I now have 60 years to live with what I learned.

1. Trust yourself: I think I knew the second I felt that lump it was cancer and thankfully I listened to my instinct that told me to go to the doctor no matter what the outcome was going to be.
2. Money cannot and will not buy happiness: I had wanted to quit my job from the second Ian was born, but I had it in my head that we needed my salary to help make us happy. I don't think we have ever been this happy and we are now on a budget.
3. Go easy on yourself: I expect way too much from myself and am my hardest critic. I learning to say no when I don't have time or I just don't want to do something. I am learning to tell myself it is okay if I am running 12 minute miles when my friend can run 8 minute miles – at least I am running.
4. Lean on God: He really does great things when you ask.
5. Use it, whatever it is: If you have something special waiting for a special occasion, use it when you feel the urge to. We had some bottles of wine Eric was holding on to and asked him why. Today is just as special a day as whatever day we are waiting for. Seriously, we never know what is going to happen and nothing is written in stone, so treat each day as special as it actually is.
6. Ask for forgiveness: Ask for forgiveness with all your heart to those you have wronged.
7. You are strong, we all are: I would have never imagined myself to be as strong as I needed to be to get through what I got through and now I see myself in a whole new light.
8. Life is special and the memories we make with each other are priceless: We can never forget we are who we are because of what we

have been through.

9. Say thank you with a smile on your face: It makes you and the person you are thanking feel great inside.

With all the memories of the past year, both good and bad, I can look at the person I am today and know in my core, it did all happen, it was all real and I wouldn't change it for the world.

More Life – October - December, 2009

Life keeps coming at us just like it always has.

October: My sister and I just got home from California visiting our family. Our grandparents are getting older and just like all the stuff I just went through, you never know what is around the next corner.

So we decided to take a few day trip out there to spend time with them.

My grandma has dementia, and we never told her about my cancer. We as a family just felt it would be too much for her to try to understand.

It was weird out there though, not talking about what had been going on was really nice.

November: I had my appointment with Dr. H yesterday; I cut right to the chase. She sat down, I told her my period was back and I was ready to talk baby talk. I was a little stunned and heartbroken after our talk.

The low down on baby #2: we have to wait until May, 2010 before we can even think about starting to try. There is no real data on the risks involved with becoming pregnant after breast cancer. Risks associated with possible reoccurrence of cancer, that is. Mainly because for the most part, those who have breast cancer were older and done with the whole kid bit. Dr. H told me she would want me to go talk to this other doctor in Dallas who dealt with fertility after breast cancer to discuss chances of cancer reoccurrence if I were to get pregnant again. It all sounded rather mind-numbing and heartbreaking to me. Truth be told, this thought has never crossed my mind. In my mind, I had cancer, I got over it, I started my period; so let's have a baby!

I guess I am still a little too la-de-da for my own good. As always, that bit of news won't stop me.

December: It is done! Shop, Sip & Share is done!

The event I have been working on for the past 2 months to benefit a local breast cancer organization. It did really well for a first time event and brought in a little over $1,600. I am very excited about this, but I also learned how hard it is to do an event like this...like REALLY hard.

Still, I must admit, I am very proud of myself for following through on this and getting it done. I have lots of ideas but once I feel overwhelmed, it is easy for me to throw in the towel and say forget it.

I do believe I have turned a whole new corner in my life with me completing this event and seeing that, yes, little steps do add up to a whole mile.

2010

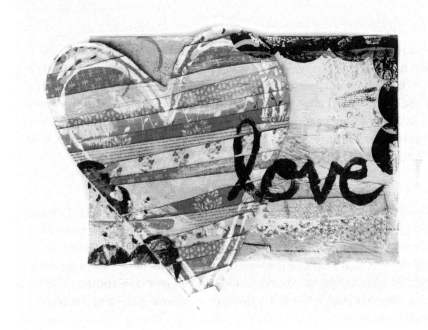

Girls can save the world – March, 2010

I noticed this saying on a shirt the other day while at one of our many play dates through the week, the little girl who wore it, was bright eyed and had a real spark for life – much like I like to think of myself as. It really made me think – girls, boys, women, men – us – we can save the world from all this drama that fills our lives daily, hourly, every second.

How do we do it – I am not sure yet, but a quote from Mahatma Gandhi has been hovering in my mind lately, "You must be the change you want to see in the world." To me this means – if we want peace, love and joy for the world, we have to be peace, love and joy. We have to live peaceful, loving, joyful lives for life itself, for human kind, for everything living – for us, for our children, for our grandchildren and so on. That means, loving people who we don't really like or agree with, giving a helping hand anytime we can, even just smiling at a stranger - we never know what his/her day has been like.

Anyway, I am not really sure where to go with this, except that we all need to know that yes, we all can save the world and more than likely it will take helping one person at a time, but we have to start somewhere – right? With that, I am putting together a card making night for a group called Cards 4 Cancer. (Side note – this used to be their blog: http://cards4cancer.wordpress.com/ but since originally writing this entry it is no longer an active website.)

I won't be able to be a part of the delivery of the cards because Eric and I will be out of town celebrating our 5th anniversary; however, I want to pour love into hand-made cards for my team to be able to deliver. It is stuff like this that I believe if we all did little tidbits here and there, this world would change, the world would grow to love one another and hate would have no choice but to be taken over by love. Eh – and the shirt would be true.

So what: - May 18, 2010

So what if I run a 12 minute mile? I can run 12 miles at a time.

So what if I don't keep a clean house? It is a home full of love and life.

So what if I can't spell? That's what spell check is four (KIDDING!!)

So what if I am an infomercial junky? I do want an easier, more exciting way to do mundane things.

So what if I get nervous in big crowds? I can still work a small one.

So what if I am a walking contradiction? I cry only to a select few.

My heart is mine to share with whom I chose. But I let small things affect my heart.

My heart is soft on the inside, but I try to make it hard on the outside; if not, I would cry for all to see.

So what if I can't organize my office? I am creative, I shouldn't be organized.

So what if I use all my cell phone minutes? I have lots of friends and family who I love and love to talk to.

So what if I get scared at home alone? That is what Eric is for, to protect me.

So what if I had cancer? Lots of good emerged, my faith, my fears, my dreams, my love for Me.

This was written sometime around November, 2010. I was training for a 1/2 marathon - it didn't happen. I did run 12 miles once. I will run 12 miles again, all of this still holds true.

Life in Cancerland - April – December, 2010

Nothing notable has happened in Cancerland for a few months, but life never stops moving.

I don't know why I am surprised by this. It seems I always am surprised at how life just keeps going though.

Eric and I went on a cruise just the two of us and it was great. We needed time to reconnect to our relationship and really celebrate what we have.

I started teaching card classes. I would make four samples of mixed media greet cards and taught the girls in my classes the techniques I used. The class made their own cards. It was a lot of work on my end – the preparation and teaching – but I loved hearing them tell me they are not creative and then by the end of the class seeing the sparkle in their eyes knowing they loved it as much as I did.

I trained for the Danskin triathlon. I was up to riding 10 miles on my bike, walking 3 miles and swimming ½ mile. This was huge for me being as I started off not being able to swim 2 laps without thinking I was about to die from lack of oxygen. I ended up pinching a nerve in my shoulder on my first and last ever open-water swim. I wasn't able to do the TRI, but I walked the last leg with a bunch of others from Team Survivor.

I potty-trained Ian. That was a lot harder than I thought it would be, but we all made it out alive.

My mom's parents both passed away within 4 months of each other. It was a hard time for us. I really started writing again during all of this.

To-do List:

Ask him about his stories
Listen to his past with undivided attention
Learn his lessons
Laugh with him
Let his laugh erupt in my ears
Hear his views
Practice his golf tips

This to-do list

was moved all around:
my calendar
my mind
my heart
now, a day late
and a dollar short
the to-do list
has faded
and can no longer be read
to him
by me
the regret in my heart
is real and heavy
and will burden my sleep

forever

Grandpa –

I love you so much and miss you with all my heart. You taught me more
than you will ever know. Most of all you taught me not to sweat the
small shit, life is too short not to be doing what I enjoy; and that I can do
anything I want to as long as I dedicate myself to it whole heartedly. ~
Enjoy your Peace in Heaven ~Good-bye...with love

Dear Grandma and Grandpa –

I miss you so much and I will never forget the love you showered us
with. I am happy y'all are together again and can be healthy and whole
in Heaven while watching over us once again. You made such a huge
impact in my life and I thank you from the bottom of my heart for all
y'all did for us grandchildren, mom, Tammy and Van. When I didn't know
where to turn, I turned to you. When I didn't know what to ask, I asked
you. When I didn't know where to go, I went to you. You were full of
love and generosity I couldn't help but learn from you. I laugh out loud
thinking of some of the things you both did - grandma, when you made
mom and grandpa split the cost of my car wreck four ways so we each
paid a fourth - no one ever thought of telling you no even though it was
my fault and I should pay for it myself. Grandpa, when you would make
us drive the white bomb just to embarrass us or your corny jokes that no
matter how many times you told them to us, we would laugh at them. I
still say some of them myself! I love you both so much and I have a void
in my heart with y'all gone but I am happy that you are no longer here in
pain and without one and other. Oh, I love you and I miss you. Until we
meet again.

I found my love for painting while taking a few on-line courses. I started
Leopards & Lilies to sell my art. Like too many other things I have started,

this one was a lot more demanding than I thought and it didn't take off as I had dreamt it would. Looking back at it though, I see I learned what I needed to from that adventure and still carry those lessons with me today. I tried to plan another Shop, Sip & Share but I just didn't have it in me. I didn't want to half ass it, so I decided it was better to cancel it. I was very sad and disappointed with myself, but I knew what was best.

Christmas came and went again. As always, we were at my sister's and had a great time. I fell down our stairs and fractured my foot, we repainted our whole down stairs (yes, we had to do this three times because I am HORRIBLE at picking out paint colors) and what looked like a nice gray looks lilac on our walls, I started teaching card making to children at our church, we went on a family cruise with Eric's family – life as I had dreamt of was ours.

2011

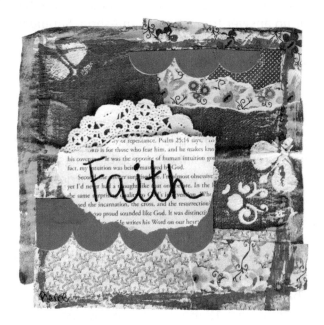

Ask and you shall receive – March 1, 2011

And no, it is not always the answer you wanted. I have still been holding on to that last prayer, that last glimmer of hope of my desire to have another child of our own. Eric on the other hand has always wanted to know the numbers.

What were my chances of getting cancer again if we did have another baby, chances after waiting three years, chances after five years, chances if we decided not to have a baby.

The problem with all this is, triple negative cancer (what I had) is a very aggressive breast cancer. There aren't a lot of numbers on life after Trip Neg because for so long, there wasn't much life after Trip Neg. It is still aggressive, but with new medicine, new ways to treat, numbers on after Trip Neg are getting better, but there still isn't much info on babies after Trip Neg.

Long story short, I have been praying for an answer, a clear black & white, yes or no answer to my heart's question. Should we ever try to have another child after I hit my 3 year mark?? I do feel in my heart this was my answer as I read a news story headline: Triple-Negative Breast Cancer risk increases with each birth.

Oh, how my heart aches with this harsh reality. But in the same breath, I have to remind myself of all the blessings we have, all of our health, our family, a life with almost no worries, family, friends, each other, and on and on and on.

Of course I still have my "wish I would have done" moments. I wish I would have tried harder to breast feed Ian. I wish I would have never gone back to work when he was 4 months because I feel I missed so much his first 18 months. I wish I would have soaked in every moment of his infancy versus waiting for the next stage and thinking that this has to get easier. But I do find comfort in knowing I held him as much I could, I loved/love him with all my heart, I kissed/kiss him as much as I could and can. I can say with 100% certainty cancer has changed my life, our family life and our future but instead of looking back on these next few years with regret about not having the family I had envisioned for us, I vow to cherish every moment, every experience and remind myself daily that life was precious and perfect even if it wasn't what I had in mind.

At least I can laugh?!?! – March 11, 2011

Today started like any other Tuesday – Ian and I were hanging out in the morning, and I was making plans for us for friend time (for both of us).

My phone rang around 9:10 and I was surprised to see Texas Oncology on my called id.

Yes, I did just have a bone and CT scan yesterday, but the results usually take a day or two.

I thought, oh they must have been super easy to read.

Nope: Dr. H wanted to see me ASAP.

Her nurse said, "Something is showing up on your scan, and she wants you in this afternoon."

I called Eric to tell him that he needed to meet me at Texas Oncology at 3:30 pm. I could barely talk to him as the words kept getting caught in my throat with the thought of what was actually happening here. Then I called Gina to tell her to come over. Once she was there, I crumbled in her arms. She tried to tell me we didn't actually know anything yet, but I knew. I always know these things. My heart knows what my head doesn't want it admit. I had a feeling when I was in the day before getting my scans that something was going to come back.

We quickly decided to go to Central Market to let the kids play while we could drink wine and zone out. We were outside eating and having a much needed glass of wine. Yes - judge away, we were there with our kids boozing it up before noon. The boys thought it would be fun to yell at the nasty birds and honestly I didn't care at that point. More than didn't care, I didn't give a fuck what others were thinking of us and our horrible parenting.

Then one lady from the other table said, "They are hurting our ears".

"Well, sorry we were here first, we sit out here for a reason, and they are just being boys," I said.

Gina and I continued to eat, the boys continued to munch on their food and run around. They started hollering down at one of our other friends who was coming up to meet us. The lady came over to us and said, "You don't own this patio."

I snapped, I was done.

"You know what, I received a call from my oncologist telling me I have cancer for a second time and at this point I don't care, I don't care what they are doing and I don't care if it is bothering you." "Well, I am on codeine, we all have our problems," was her smug response.

Then me and Gina just laughed, we can't help it we just laughed. I wish I was on codeine! My other friend got there at the very tail end of the "confrontation" and Gina and I were laughing and crying. She had no idea what is going on and I just wanted to drink more wine.

And that we did. I went and bought us another bottle of wine. We sat out in the sunshine, laughed together, cried together and enjoyed ourselves. It was now time. I had to face the music of my unknown fate. I had to get going to see Dr. H.

Eric came home to pick me up to take me to Dr. H's office. After getting there, I was now afraid I might puke from the little bit of too much wine and my nerves were wrecked. Eric and I tried to pass time by playing each other in *Words with Friends*. I guess it helped the puking feeling. Then there it was. It was my name being called by the nurse. I held on to Eric's hand to steady myself from the wine or the nerves. I can't tell the difference at this point. Shit here we go is all I could think. Knock, knock we heard on the door. Fuck, it is real, flooded my mind. "Hi there, can I come in," she asked. I wanted to say no, but instead I said yes. "So, have you been feeling okay lately" and right then I knew. "Well, I have been having trouble breathing but I thought it was seasonal allergies."

You thought wrong sucker that nagging little voice in me said. She said there was a chance it was some random infection to which I said, "well a child in Ian's mother day out had whooping cough." "Have you had a cough?" she asked. "No," I replied, "Not whooping cough…" Yes, I was grasping for anything. Anything but what I knew was coming next.

From this point on, I am not really sure what was said…I went to that place I seem to go to when I am receiving horrible news.

Two masses on my lungs, one on each; might be wrapped around a blood vessel and lymph node, some smaller areas of concern on bones.

She told me we couldn't know it was cancer until we had gathered all our facts, which would be in my lung biopsy.

Here is what I did hear though: the sadness in her voice when she told me to gather my support system because I was going to need them; the love in her hug as I broke down and sobbed in her arms. Somehow, I pulled it together enough to walk out of her office down to the scheduling area. We left, holding hands, united as one. Once again I had no idea who to call or what to do. So we sat in the car and cried. We now knew we must do something because this wasn't going away. I called mom, asked her if she could talk. I was a puddle on the phone and probably didn't make much sense. I texted Gina and asked her to invite the girls over at 8:30 after the kids were down. Eric and I made margaritas and let Ian eat dinner on the couch. Girls arrived promptly at 8:30. Wine drinking started right away and went on for a while, a long while.

Wednesday: I woke up pretty hung over. I rallied, got ready, made Ian's lunch, hung out with the boys and hit the road. I forgot how much I hate morning traffic (one of the many perks of my life). I finally got to the lung doctor after getting lost a few times. I had to take too many breathing tests and then I waited. He came in, we talked and I decided he was a cool guy and I know why Dr. H sent me to him. He knew his stuff and was bad ass at what he did. He told his nurse to clear his schedule for Friday which of course made my heart beat a little faster. We talked some more about the procedure and scheduled the bronchoscope for Friday. Although I heard what he said, I was still clueless as to what I would be having done. I left thinking this isn't really happening. How can this really be happening? I went to the library, lunch, to pick up Ian, hang out at home for an hour or so and then I was off to have a brain MRI.

I was tired of being poked at this point. Two pokes later and I had yet another IV this week. MRI is nothing exciting and although the knocking was random and odd, I found it a little soothing. I think this shows how stressed I was at this point. At 6:30 pm the oncologist called to tell me my brain was good!! WHOOP WHOOP, one for Team S.

Thursday: Normal day around here. Ian had his swim lessons, I went to the gym with Gina, we all met for lunch at Phil's Ice House, home to hang out and play. I finally looked online and decided I needed collective prayers for a lung fungus, sent out the word for that to be the prayer. My Mom and Rachele thought I was a little strange but said they would go along with my plan – thanks y'all!!

Friday: Ugh, here we go. We got up trying to keep this like a normal day. We all got ready and then took Ian over to a friend's house. We got to the hospital got checked in and were taken back to my room. I had to get poked again – TWO times if you were wondering. IV count for the week: THREE. Eric and I hung out, people were in and out to talk to us, the doctor was in, the drugs were in and I was out. Once I woke up, I willed myself to wake more up because at this point I was ready to go home and be done. I asked the nurse if I could look at her Cooking Light magazine, because who doesn't like to look at yummy food when you know you can't eat? I was wheeled back to my room where Eric was waiting for me and, after I told him I was looking at the magazine, he said, "We can get the cooking channel again."

And right then I knew the answer to my question.

"What is it?"

"Is it?"

"Yes"

"FUCK" I seemed to be using this word a lot lately.

We talked about what the doctor told him. It was small (under 1 cm) and seemed to be in only one spot. My doctor came in and explained a little more of what he found. I still was not 100% sure if the spot was in a lymph node or right by it – eh, I'll find out soon enough. I had to hear all the warnings about coughing up blood, high temp, blah, blah, blah. I was ready to blow this joint. At 3:00pm – I could FINALLY drink some water and eat. I thought I was to about to dry up. By 3:30pm – We picked up Ian, headed home for a *normal* night.

Three Little Words – March 15, 2011

You have cancer

WHAT THE F*CK!?!?

Remember to breathe.

It's breast cancer.

It is small.

It's stage one.

Whole world spins

chemo, surgery, radiation.

You're done!

Celebrate, cheer, love!

One year goes by,

you're still clean!

Two years later,

you look great!

Approaching 3 years...

off the anti-depressants...

Abnormal CT scan...

F*CK F*CK F*CK!!!

In the lungs

All is unknown...

scared, pissed, sad...

Ready to fight!

Be bald again.

Ask for help.

Ask for prayers...

Cry, laugh, love.

Tailspin – March 19, 2011

The world as we knew it was promptly busted around 9:45am Friday morning. The results were in from the tumor biopsy. I felt like someone punched me in the stomach and kicked me in the ribs while I was down and then pulled my hair just for fun. *I HAVE STAGE IV METASTATIC BREAST CANCER.* What this means is, it is the same cancer as in the breast, it has moved to my lungs and 3 spots in some bones and ribs. I'm not really sure of all the details because as soon as I heard the words "treatable but not curable" I pretty much floated into a bubble and only heard tidbits of information. I now know how Charley Brown felt all those years – you are there, you know something is being said but you can't for the life of you focus, listen and hear.

We are looking into MD Anderson to see if there is a clinical trial for me to be in and if not I will start chemo within two weeks. And within these two weeks, I will have to go to day-surgery to get a port. Eric still has many questions as to the treatment(s) so we still aren't sure what exactly is going to be happening. I do know this, it is going to be a long road, it is going to be hard but it is all going to be worth every second of the hard work to get to live this wonderful life with my hubby, Ian, family and friends. I can't thank everyone enough for the loving emails, texts and voicemails. I am not ready to talk about this yet and honestly, I am not sure I ever will be. To me it is what it is, we are going to do what needs to be done and our *normal* life will now just be a different level of normal.

The wind storm – March 21, 2011

How do you stay still in the middle of a wind storm? I am not sure.

"I cannot change the direction of the wind, but I can adjust my sails to always reach my destination."- Jimmy Dean

Eric and I were sitting on the couch while my mom and Marci were fluttering about cleaning and organizing our house (because lets be real, some things I am not good at) and he said, I guess this is something we need to get used to....sitting still while others aren't. I asked how we keep still in the middle of a wind storm. "Get to the middle...the center of a tornado is still" he replied. So, how do we as a family get to the middle of the tornado, hunker down and stay still?

At church yesterday, our pastor preached about claiming our wholeness. He explained there are two perceptions when we think of asking for things. We feel 100% different about asking our boss for a raise and not knowing what the answer will be versus when our boss asks us to do a project for him and we already know what the answer will be. The point was when I, we, everyone prays, I shouldn't ask for me to be healed, cured, fixed (yes, I feel broken), etc. I need to know I am already whole and healed in His eyes and I need to pray this way. I need to pray from a place where I am already cured, where I am already free of disease, where I am already with my son who is grown and I was there to see it all happen.

What I ask of you is to pray from a place of gratitude, grace and light. Don't pray from a place of desperation, fear and anger. Don't pray: Dear God, please let me have a healthy pregnancy. Instead pray, Dear God, thank You for my healthy baby. For me I pray, Dear God, thank You for my healthy body and every little cell being well. Thank You for the long life ahead of me full of love, laughter and light.

"You must take personal responsibility. You cannot change the circumstances, the season, or the wind, but you change yourself. That is something you are in charge of." – Jim Rohn

I am trying….trying as hard as I can to find this place, to know I am in charge of me, my thoughts, my love for myself and others, my everything. I am trying to find my middle safe place but man alive, right now I do feel like I have been sucked up into the tornado and am flying around with the cows.

Scared….shitless – March 22, 2011

"You gain strength, courage, and confidence by every experience in which you really stop to look fear in the face. You must do something which you think you cannot do." – Eleanor Roosevelt.

Now, I am NOT saying I can't and won't beat this, but I am scared shitless at this point in time. We listened to the meeting with Dr. H from Friday when we found out the *news*. I heard things I worked really hard to forget (yes maybe by drinking lots of wine) during the weekend. I made another appointment with her yesterday for today because we had time to get our heads on straight, think rationally and ask coherent questions (Friday….not so much). So we now know the following things are for sure – whereas Friday we were kind of sure, maybe, not really. The main spot on my lung is kind of in the middle of my chest and is about 2 inches. We can't biopsy more now from this spot because it is in front of my heart and well at this point a needle in my heart isn't going to help matters much.

There are several (still not sure HOW many) spots IN my lungs (before I was thinking they were on my lungs...not sure why) and each of these is about the size of pea. We can't do surgery on these because they are small and randomly all over the place. I am still not 100% sure about the bone...it is in my bones but barely because it did NOT register on the bone scan. It is on a rib and in my left shoulder area.

Eric then wanted to have a private conversation with Dr. H which I was fine with. Not really sure what all was said and at this point I don't care. My mind is made up that I don't care...I don't care what is said, I am going to be here...for my life, for Eric, for Ian, for my family, for my friends...I DON'T CARE what they say. I DON'T F-IN CARE!!!

I asked for a 3 week plan. (I think I like figuring out steps in 3 weeks at a time – less than a month but manageable.) First, get an appointment with MD Anderson in Houston, go get thrown through a gamut of tests again, figure out if they have any trials going on that would benefit me – if yes, great – go to Houston once a week. If no, see what they would recommend. If same as Dr. H, get treatment here. If different, figure out what is different, have them collaborate and see what option is better. How we are going to actually make this decision – I have no idea. Eric found several other trials throughout the country that we were hoping would pan out to be something....but unfortunately they did not. SO pretty much, in 3 weeks I will be on chemo. If we go with Dr. H my treatment will be weekly infusion for 3 weeks on and 1 week off for 5 – 10 months. "A coward gets scared and quits. A hero gets scared, but still goes on." – Anonymous

I came up with my new prayer: Thank You God for my body which is a vessel of radiant health that is full of life, love, laughter and light for at least another 50 years. I am scared...very scared.

The panic – March 27, 2011

When it hits,

it hits hard and fast.

It likes to come at the oddest times,

unloading the dishwasher,

reading an innocent text,

in the middle of church.

When it sneaks in a little,

I can put it back where it belongs,

in the trash,

not in my heart,

not in my head.

But when it attacks,

 hard and fast

my defenses are down,

it gets in but only for a minute,

only for a few tears,

only for a few panicked breaths of fear of hate of rage.

Peace!

Be still,

I muster inside,

in my mind,

then my heart

and panic knows

it is not welcome here.

Not now,

not ever!

The Talk – March 28, 2011

We all know as parents and children having talks with our parents and/or children that we do NOT want to have are inevitable...the dreaded *sex* talk. The *you aren't doing so well in school* talk. The *I am pretty sure who you are dating is a loser* talk. Everyone is uncomfortable, no one wants to talk about it, but at some point the parent has to suck it up and do it. I would rather have 100 *sex* talks than the talk we need to have with Ian. Hell, I would rather have the *sex* talk with my grandparents rather than our talk that is looming over our heads and in our hearts. We are trying to figure out the right timing. Timing with a 3 year old is everything. When Eric gets home, Ian is not in listen mode. I can't have the talk by myself because even when I have the talk in my head, I break down.

WHEN are we going to do this? We went to this place today called Wonders & Worries. They are an awesome group who will have play therapy sessions with Ian for at least 6 weeks to make sure he is processing this and is able to express his feelings. But in the meantime, it is up to us...to tell him, "Mommy has cancer." How do we explain to him what cancer is when I still can't wrap my head around it? How do we tell him what I am going to be like during chemo? Tired and blah but still his mommy who loves him more than anything and wants so bad to be the one who is able to take care of him? How do we tell him we aren't sure how long this is going to last? How do we tell him any of this sh*t, any of this that no child should ever hear, much less a 3 year old? Today was a really hard day for both me and Eric. Visiting that place and then getting my scheduled appointment at MD Anderson on Friday totally solidified this...it is happening, it is real, it is about to begin. Life as we know it might never return, and my heart hurts.

Mr. Science Guy – March 30, 2011

I am losing my ability to make decisions – any decision. I have been looking at Eric to help me with decisions because in my mind he is Mr. Science Guy. I feel two things with this loss of decision making and leaning on Eric more – I feel like a part of me is gone because I have never been so needy but on the other hand I feel stronger for recognizing that I need help and asking for it and finally, accepting it!

Loving What Is – April 4, 2011

After visiting with my pastor a few weeks ago he recommended I read a book called "Loving What Is" by Byron Katie. It is a very interesting book and really solidified my belief in my thought of - it is what it is. She says in the book there are three types of business: your own business, someone else's business or God's business. When you are in someone else's business you cannot be totally whole and present in your own business. Example: you are all up in a friend's business in what your friend shouldn't have done in some situation – none of your business. You can't be present in your own business if you are wrapped up in someone else's business. I am looking at my health as God's business. It is His to take control of, it His to do with what He needs to do, it is His – not mine.

One of my best friends told me today at the gym that she doesn't understand how I am handling this so well. In my mind, there is nothing for me to handle. Yes it sucks big time that I will be in chemo for maybe 10 months or maybe 10 years. At this point I don't know. But I do know that no amount of worry, no amount of "what if" scenarios played out in my mind, no amount of anything but putting one foot in front of the other will help me right now. Now, don't get me wrong. I have major breakdowns, I get pissed, I really want to beat up a fax machine with a baseball bat and listen to "Damn it feels good to be gangster" (little Office reference if you didn't get it). I do give myself a few minutes daily. Not a few hours, not a few days...only a few minutes of my pissed pity party and then I have to gather myself again and move on.

I had one of those today when I was trying to decide what day I should have chemo. I just needed to know what days after chemo I would feel my worst, and no one could seem to tell me. I was mad. Someone just tell me something so I can know what to do. After talking to a great friend who also works at Texas Oncology I got my answer. She asked the pharmacist and, according to him, 90% of people just felt really worn down but not down and out like I was last time. Eric did a little more research and I am thinking I will feel like I have a cold. No one day seems to be worse than another. That is what I needed to know. I just needed some facts. If all goes as planned my first chemo day will be this Friday at 10 am.

"Life is full of ups and downs. The trick is to enjoy the ups and have courage during the downs." - Anonymous

The truth of the matter – April 7, 2011

"You never find yourself until you face the truth" – Pearl Bailey

Today has been a big fat ugly rollercoaster of emotions that I was stuffing way down deep until I talked to my dad. My dad is a man of very few words but it takes people like that to really get to me because I know what he is saying is from the heart and he isn't just talking to talk. There was just something about him telling me he would take my place in a second if he could that crumbled my wall I had been hiding behind. It hit me and hit me hard, I was scared. I didn't want to start chemo tomorrow or ever. I didn't want this. I didn't ask for it and I didn't want it. But then in my next breath I looked at my sweet angel Ian and knew it didn't matter what I asked for because this was what I had and I would do anything in my power to live for him, for Eric, for myself – anything.

After lunch I had to head to my obstetrician's office for a quick check up before starting chemo. This really hit me hard seeing other happy pregnant women in there. I was so very envious of them, of their lives, of what I would never have again: a pregnant belly with a life inside me. It would take all I had to hold onto this life inside of me right now. I was scared but I was alive.

I don't want to start chemo but it will save me. I don't want to have cancer but it will guide me to be someone bigger and better than I am. I guess the simplest version of the truth of my matter right now is, I am living and will continue to be for a very long time. Maybe I will be on chemo, maybe not but there is only one way to figure it out –START!

Chemo Chronicle 2.1 – April 9, 2011

Today started like any other day – Ian woke up at 6:40am and needed me to come lay with him. Of course I can't refuse when we got to snuggle in his bed and chit chat for 20 minutes until his star goes off. 9:20am came fast but slow. Time seems to be a weird thing lately. It has been exactly one month since I received the call about an abnormal CT scan. Since that Tuesday so much has happened – tests, biopsy, MD Anderson, visits from best friend, family, a few break downs and normal days in between.

In one way I felt like I should have started chemo forever ago but on the hand I couldn't believe I was already starting – crazy. Kissing Ian good-bye this morning was like a kick to the gut (really, I don't know what that is like because I have never been in a fight in my life. Except on little altercation with a best friend but that was just me pulling her hair. Oh and that one time I *might* have hit a boyfriend with a car – that is still up for debate as well. So all in all, I have never actually been hit! I digress, back to today). Pulling into the Texas Oncology garage was when it hit - the sick feeling in my stomach, the wonder of how I was going to make it up the stairs, the fear of what was about to happen to me and what my body was doing to itself. I had to get blood drawn today – d*mn it! Two pokes later, they had the blood. After that I decided I AM getting a port...sometime next week. My veins suck (not due to this crap, they just always have) and if I needed blood and an IV every Friday – well that just wasn't happening.

After talking with the nurse practitioner, Eric remembered to ask her about my side. I THOUGHT I had gotten a few spider bites on my right side right under my ribs and all who know me know that is the way I react to any kind of bite. It was no surprise that I thought this major swelling around the bites was just spider bites....it isn't spider bites. (No it isn't the cancer trying to come out of my skin, either – hey, a girl can hope!) I have shingles... WTF?!?! I guess this virus is in most of us if we had chicken pox and then it likes to come out when there is a change in stress level – NO idea what brought on the change of stress level!! Okay, now I know I have shingles, was armed with a load of prescriptions we were off to the infusion room. Nothing too exciting happened here. It took about 2 hours in the infusion, but it won't take that long once I get my port. After we got home, I passed out for about an hour and a half, got up felt great, went to Chuy's for dinner because that just sounded really good – and it was!

Everyone wants to know how I feel. I feel fine – tired but fine. I am curious to see what the next few days bring?

Hungry – April 10, 2011

Last night, at dinner with Eric, listening to live music, celebrating our 6th anniversary, we (or maybe I) launched into the conversation of 6 years ago...We had NO idea where our lives would be today, would Eric have still married me knowing I was riddled with cancer (yes, I can be a TAD dramatic) and of course he being the prince he is said, "First off, you are NOT riddled with cancer. Second, you couldn't have stopped me from marring you." Oh I do love him.

As most dinners go with a glass of wine, the "why" of it all came up. I said, "I just wish I knew my reason for this – I know there is a reason but what is it?" *Would I do something different if I knew my reason for this? Is my reason for this really for me? What if it is to affect someone else to cause them to do something great – who knows? I would love to know.* Eric had a great response though – you are never greater at what you are doing than while you are hungry for the outcome. Once you get to the outcome - your ultimate goal, you let your guard down, you stop trying as hard as you once were because you are there. This all made me really think. *What would I do now if I knew my ultimate reason? Would I try as hard as I am now to understand it – I don't know...why would I if I already understood it?* So it brings me back to my question of, "what is my reason for this?" I really wish I knew but I am not sure I will ever know. I guess it goes back to everyone's question – what is our purpose here on earth...I want to think it is to love each other unconditionally but I am sap. For now, I will stay hungry for life, love, a cure, my purpose, joy, happiness, my family & friends and so much more.

Dear Cancer.... – April 13, 2011

Unfortunately we meet again. I beat you last time and I will beat you this time as well. I still don't understand you, I have no love nor hate for you. I just ask God every day that you go away from me, from everybody...forever. What is it about life that you want to take away from me, from so many? Well the joke is on you cancer. You will be taken out when you are least expecting it. You will be imploded in my body, in whoever's body you are trying to take over – you will not survive. If there was a deal to make – eat only one thing for the rest of my life, walk on my hands, run 10 miles a days – I would do it. I would do it in a heartbeat. It would take every ounce of faith I had to trust you though....if we made a deal. You aren't very trustworthy.

Cancer, don't you get it? You are in a body that has a three and a half year old son, a wonderful husband, is a daughter, a sister, a friend and so much more. Don't you get it – you are not welcome here. Nobody wants you here in my body or in any body's body. Everybody you are in has a life outside of you. Everybody you are in is something to someone else. You try to make yourself their, my, our lives, but you can't. You are not my life. You are a part of my life right now, but not for long. You will never be my life. If you are trying to fit in with the crowd you are going about all the wrong way. You get way more friends with honey than vinegar. Why don't you try that – why don't you try being nice and see where that gets you. You can't like what you are. You can't be proud of what you are. You can better. It is never too late to change. I will even offer to help you change; to be better, to stop this downward spiral you are in....I will help you. I am ready to start helping you whenever, now, yesterday – the sooner the better.

Sincerely,

Renee

Bittersweet – April 14, 2011

I try to shut out the bitter in my *oh so sweet* moments of the day. But it is hard. I try to hand all the bitter over to God but a little is left on my fingers. I try to remember that five good days out of seven is a great percentage. I try to remember friends having babies is a miracle although not mine. I try to remember normal has changed several times before and doesn't mean it can't go back. I try to remember a time when cancer wasn't in my vocabulary in my life. I try to remember my determination is strong, my love for life is stronger, my spirit is strongest. I try to remember these oh so sweet times.

Chemo Chronicle 2.2 – April 15, 2011

Of course today started early at 6:40am – why does Ian's internal clock go off at 6:40am no matter what time he goes to bed?!?! Got to Texas Oncology, checked in, blood drawn (ONE STICK TODAY!!!), vitals checked and good to go. Talked to Dr. H's nurse practitioner, my blood levels were fabulous, she told me I COULD take TWO Aleve at a time for bone pain (YIPPIE!!), we talked about a test they sent my tumor to have – pretty much DNA testing on my tumor and it came back with which chemos it WOULD respond to and I was on one of the three that it WOULD respond to!! Dr. H stepped in to say hi and to check on me. (Yes, I do love my oncologist!) We chatted about a friend of mine I met through the pink ribbon cowgirls who was diagnosed in November as Stage IV right off the bat – her last PET scan – NADA – all disease is gone. I told Dr. H I heard what she did for her and I was shooting for clean PET scan in 6 months.

They laughed and called me an overachiever but to hear Dr. H tell me she had big plans for me and she was ready to knock this sh*t out of the park – made my heart smile. NOW that was what I was talking about!! I did find it very interesting though when I sat down to do my nightly writing I found a book Eric's sisters, mom and GG got me "God's Inspirational Promises." I opened it up and it landed on the page about courage. The message was "the disciples were common men given a compelling task. Before they were the stained glass saints, they were somebody's next-door-neighbors trying to make a living and raise a family. There weren't cut from theological cloths or raised on supernatural milk. But they were an ounce more devoted than they were afraid and, as a result, did some extraordinary things." Again, just what I needed to hear tonight. They were people, like you and me....simple as that. All it takes is a little courage and miracles are possible. Yes, I am holding out for my miracle and I feel it in my being that it is there ready to be had.

A dream team – April 17, 2011

In church today we had a WONDERFUL message: building your dream team. It started with a little insight about geese flying in a V and why they do what they do. It was all very interesting; by flying in a V formation they get 71% less wind resistance than if they flew solo. They honk at the one in front to give encouragement and when the one in front gets tired, he goes to the back. How amazing is that? I think it is very interesting!

Then we had a guest speaker: Mindy Audlin. She was talking about building a dream team and how even Jesus needed a dream team so who are we to think we can do this all on our own?? I feel like I have a dream team behind me for this go around. Now, don't get me wrong – I had support the first go around but only the support I allowed in...and it wasn't much only because I was stubborn (I know, me stubborn?!?!) This time, I don't have a choice – my neighborhood honeys (who are MUCH more than other mommies that I hang out with all the time – they have become best friends) they won't let me tell them no, they won't let me hole up and be sad, they won't let me be on a team by myself. And let me tell you, I feel stronger than ever with my dream team behind me every step of the way. Oh, back to church...she then told us to ask one another these two questions: What is it you feel you are being called to do? And what do you need to get it done? I feel I am called to help people communicate with each other, spread love and joy to each other, and enhance each other's lives. I am working on this – I have a wonderful idea that I am getting together and am almost ready to share. What do I need to get it done? Well, first and foremost to find the courage to step out and do it (and I feel me writing it here will do just that).

Then after I create what I need to create I need help marketing it. It is scary to step out and talk about this dream; it is scary to think what I would do if it took off but oh so exciting. It is scary to think that I would need to do it on my own, but then I remember there is no way I have to do anything on my own – all we have to do is ask.

But, seriously, what NOT to say to someone with cancer - April 20, 2011

I was texting Gina last night and told her my hair was starting to fall out. Her response was so pure and honest, "I don't know what to say," she texted me. "I don't know what to say" – what a great thing to say when in fact you don't know what to say. Instead of saying something that makes you feel better, you say the truth... the truth that you don't know what in the hell to say. Why is it so hard for us, as people, as friends, as family to be 100% honest with each other? Hey, I am 100% guilty of this as well. I will tell 98% of the truth when asked how I feel, when asked personal things. I don't know why. I think we are scared to be judged by others (of course we are, we all love to judge each other). Or more so, we are scared that if we tell the whole truth, then when our situation changes, the person we told the whole truth to will still remember the whole truth and be in the past moment instead of in the present with what is happening now.

I know people are coming from a good place and everyone truly wants to be a good friend, but....

A few others things we people with cancer do NOT want to hear from you are:

Oh, so and so was cured at MD Anderson (or some other *hot* place to go). YES, some people go to different places and have great responses, but we all need to remember everybody's story is different.

You don't know what type of cancer that person had, you have no idea what type of cancer...there are so many variables involved.

Oh, so and so went through chemo and it was a breeze or it was horrible. Again, not something anyone who is going to start chemo wants to hear because it makes their fight seem like is it supposed to be a breeze.

When one door closes another door opens. . Again, we with the cancer know this and do not feel it your place to tell us. Your health closing the door on you is NOT the time to throw out this little ditty.

God never gives you more than you can handle. Really?!?!? Come on. We all know what we can and can't handle, we know God in our own way and don't need you telling us this.

Saying "you poor thing" don't give a pity look or "OMG THAT IS HORRIBLE" look either because I guarantee the person telling you this news KNOWS this is horrible and doesn't need to read it on your face.

Why are you so tired? Well, because my body is being bombarded by chemo, which yes is to save my life, but also takes a slight toll on me physically.

Are you going to wear a wig? NO – losing my hair is the least of my worries and if you need me to have a wig to make you feel better about the situation. Unfortunately, I feel too many wear wigs to make others feel more comfortable.

Chemo Chronicle 2.3 – April 22, 2011

I wish I could say, "Third time's the charm" – hardly. More like
3 strikes and you are OUT! I had never had this much pain from
a port access and I pray to never have it again. I am still super
swollen from the port surgery on Tuesday, but it all still SUCKED big
time.

My nurse poked me once and hit the side of the port. She poked
me twice and hit the side of the port again...this lead into my first
breakdown of the day. I couldn't help it; the tears came out of
nowhere and wouldn't stop. I couldn't even look at her when she
left the room. I felt like a baby, I felt bad for making her feel bad
and at this point I was already done with the day and ready to go
home. She knew I was done and said she would get someone else.

The next RN came in, talked to me, had me lay down and got it –
thank goodness. It wasn't like the poke hurt - it was the pressure
they had to apply to the actual port that hurt like hell. Dr. H came
in, looked at this lovely rash I had on my chest and a little around
my mouth, gave me some steroid cream, told me it wouldn't grow
hair on my chest (THANKS!) and then left.

We sat in the waiting area for at least an hour before they told me
my blood counts were low and were waiting to hear from Dr. H. I
was so frustrated and if it wasn't for Erica, I might have screamed.
She is so great at what she does and finally got them to tell me
what in the hell was the hold up. All I needed to know was Dr. H
was in one room this whole time. I get it, I want an hour with her
if I need an hour and I love that she spends the time needed with
each patient. I just needed to be told this today. Instead I sat out
there thinking my name got lost in the shuffle and just kept getting
passed up. I finally get called to go back to the chemo room, get a
chair but still wasn't told about Dr. H being with the same patient
nor what was actually up with my blood. There are several factors

that could have been off with my blood. Then sitting there, I had another breakdown or two or three...I lost count! I felt lost in the sea of other patients, I felt powerless and out of control. I was SO SO SO thankful to have Eric there with me. He went to ask what was up and that is when we were finally told she had been in one room the whole time. They also told him it was my white blood count that was at 1.2 and anything below 1.5 is iffy.

Finally Dr. H gave the go ahead for me to get chemo. I will get a neulasta shot on Monday. SH*T, I don't want this shot. It makes my bones hurt so flipping bad, or at least it did last time. Anyway, once I was hooked up chemo was a breeze; I worked on necklaces and watched TV. I tried so hard to be centered, to get back to level ground while I was breaking down but I couldn't. I couldn't get the negative out and the peace back in – goes to show me I have A LOT of work to do with being at peace with this, with everything. So all in all today sucked but picking up Ian was like a breath of fresh air. And I am SO glad next week is an off week....I need a week off from this bullsh*t.

Honestly – April 25, 2011

I honestly had a horrible day today. I sat in my car and cried: cried for me; cried for the fact that Eric and Ian are going to shave my head tonight; cried because we now really have to tell Ian something (or why in the hell would I let him help shave my head?); cried because my stomach hurts from the laxatives I have to take; cried because chemo is already shutting down my ovaries and with that brings much heartache...no hormones means NO hormones and NO of a lot that a healthy 32 year old woman should be; cried because my mom and Gina's husband both told me how beautiful I am bald...I just cried. All of this happened before I willed myself to walk up the two flights of stairs to get a shot that I didn't want and while I sat in the waiting area I ate a nasty cup of soup from Whole Foods because I needed comfort and I didn't want to call anyone because I honestly didn't want to talk about it. Laurie had even texted me to ask if I was okay because I had been on her mind. Yes, I do believe God was sending me an angel at that moment but I wasn't ready to except His helping hand.

Even though I didn't accept God's help with Laurie; He was persistent and sent me Sarah while I was waiting for my shot. Oh how I needed Sarah! She has been through this sh*t twice BUT they (her hubby and her) just had a baby from a surrogate with their own embryo – AWESOME! I needed her. I needed someone who understood why my bones hurt and just how they feel when they do hurt, I needed to talk to her, to see her sweet baby, to give her a hug of friendship and survivorship. I needed her. I have no wise closing, no clever saying I just have honesty from me to you on this day.

Finding Renee: - April 27, 2011

She was buried way down deep. The light was almost burnt out, but God kept fanning it, even when she didn't. She was tired of telling herself no. She was tired of making excuses. She was tired of not trying. She was tired of tired. She knew the day was here she had no choice but to do what she was being called to do. She had no choice but to start believing in her own self. She had no choice but to say yes – to herself, to life, to God.

I found a whole file of poems and stuff I wrote the last go around with "this" that I was too afraid to post. I am not sure why I was afraid or why I didn't, but I didn't. I am going to now. I am going to put it all out there to help me heal, to help you, to help God work through me, just to help. I really feel like I need to help. Help who? I'm not sure. It is too easy to go back to that place of "I am not organized enough" or "How can I pull this off" or "Who am I to think this is a good idea" and so many more. I am slowly learning. Who cares that I am not organized to on lookers. I am organized in myself.

Good-bye hair – April 28, 2011

Well, we did it. I sat in a chair out on the back porch while Eric shaved my head and Ian played with his bubbles from the Easter bunny. He couldn't have cared less what was happening with my hair. It is funny though. It made me realize the things that are such big deals to adults usually don't matter at all to children. Maybe we should take cues from children. They are true masters of being in the moment and knowing what truly is important. I am "assuming" that in Ian's eyes nothing with me has changed. I am still his mommy who snuggles with him every morning and tells him "No, you cannot jump off the fifth stair up" a few times every day. It wasn't as big of a deal as I thought it would be. It was nothing like last time.

Last time we shaved my head I had lots of people over for a head shaving party. In hind sight I am not sure why. Maybe I didn⍰t want to be alone with what was happening? This time, I wanted it to be just us 3, the core of me. I was very blasé about it. It was what needed to be done, and I am so glad it is now done. I do remember how wearing a scarf makes me feel like I have cancer. To me, it is screams, ⍰I HAVE CANCER!⍰ I am working on being comfortable with not wearing anything on my head outside our house. It is hard though. Those looks, those looks of pity tear into my soul. I don␟t want pity, I want a *HELL YEAH you rock* or a *F*CK cancer sucks*; something, anything other than pity. So here it is... me sans hair. This is me. This is who I will be for an uncertain amount of time but I am okay with it. My hair didn't define me and now my lack of won't either.

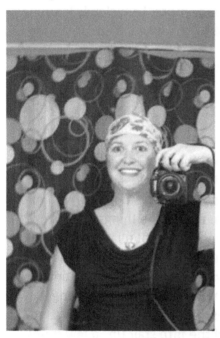

Unconditional Love - April 30, 2011

It really hit me Sunday while sitting at first service and seeing it more crowded than I have ever seen it before and hearing them say that Easter is hands down the busiest service of the year. It hit me hard the unconditional love God has for us. He sent us Jesus to teach us one thing – unconditional love. He made it look so simple. Have an open heart, an open mind and love for all, but we as humans make it so hard on ourselves. We (and yes I am included in this "we") like to put conditions on our love to others, to ourselves, even to God.

I would love my co-worker if she would listen to me. I would love the homeless man on the street if he would get a job. I will love myself when I lose those last 5 pounds. I will be happy when I get a promotion. I will love God again after He gives me a baby. Even though you are a miracle worker and have saved 1,000 of people's lives, I can't love you wholly because you are Jewish, or some other religion. I will love my husband more once he tells me how pretty I am.

Do you see how ridiculous all these sound? Do you see how many conditions are put on something so simple, so available to us at all times? If we just look in our hearts and see what God gave us, the ability to love unconditionally like He Loves us. But we don't. We line up our love and dole it out to those we think deserve it. But the catch is, we deserve love from every person and every person deserves our love. I mean all of it, not a little snip of it when it is convenient for us, not a little piece of it when we feel like it. Every person deserves all of our love all of the time.

Try to love someone today that you might not any other day. If they aren't there for you to show a kind smile to, give a gentle pat on the back then think of them. Think of them with loving thoughts and send them love from your heart. It will make you feel amazing. Just try it.

But, what is right??? – May 4, 2011

Taken from the lesson at church on Sunday: Our pastor posed the question or statement to us; however you chose to look at it. What is right with the world? What IS right with the world. It is easy to launch into all the horrible things that are happening around the world, but if we stop to really look at the outcome of these events it is nothing short of a miracle that is taking place. Japan for example, they have people all over the world praying for them, they have people all over the world donating money to them, they have people working together to help them be able to help themselves, they have support, love and light being sent to them 24 hours a day. What a miracle is that? How easy it is for people to pull together when need be. In my opinion we should pull together like that when there isn't a tragedy but we can take it one step at a time!

Look at my situation. I have people all over the place praying for me, my family, for us. The net of love that has been thrown around us is so strong, thick and tight it is unbreakable. People I haven't talked to in years contributed to a care package one of my good friends put together for us. Not only did they send me loving cards of encouragement, they sent them to Eric and fun gifts for Ian. Yes, he thought the Easter bunny showed up early!! Another friend of mine, Tarah, coordinated and made a quilt out of squares of fabric that were sent to her by some of my high school friends and family. It was incredible reading what they wrote to me, the inspiration and love they sent to me. I cried from the love I felt in their words. So what is right with my world: God, life, love, family, friendship, my desire to smile from my heart, my urge to create and write, my longing to help others, and so much more! It is too easy to get trapped in our thoughts of what is wrong but we can look at the same situation and say what is right just as easily as saying what is wrong.

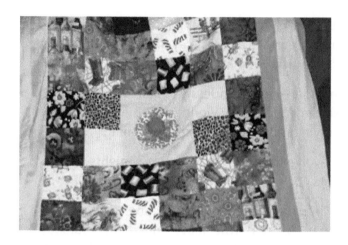

Thursdays – May 5, 2011

Thursdays have evolved for me over time. Before Ian, Thursday meant one day away from the weekend, one day away from getting to just hang out. Many years ago, we had a girl's poker night every other Thursday night. I am not really sure why we ever thought doing this on a Thursday night was a good idea because we all still had to work on Friday. Well every other Thursday night, we didn't take anything seriously except hanging out with the 6 of us, drinking entirely too much wine, smoking an unknown number of cigarettes between the 6 of us, and asking the pizza delivery guy to go buy us more beer, wine or cigarettes. We were at least smart enough to know we shouldn't be driving and occasionally we would take the poker game at hand a little too serious but not often. Oh these Thursday nights meant so much to us. Some of us didn't know each other when we started this get together. Some of us were already great friends, but at those poker nights we really opened up to each other and became so much more than the poker girls.

Now that was just poker nights, Laurie and I had many other Thursday night happy hour(s). Let's just say after 4 hours of happy hour, Eric would come pick us up and deliver us home safely.

Then there was the apartment with Jessica - balcony, wine, and music. We were settled in for many wonderful Thursday nights of talking, laughing, crying, singing...you name, we did it.

Life was bound to evolve from the crazy Thursday nights to the more sensible nights.

Ian was born and Thursday nights now meant one more day until Eric was home with us. My maternity leave ended and Thursday nights turned into only 6 more hours of work until I get to be with Ian and Eric all day.

Once again life has evolved and with it my Thursdays have too. The days bring complete happiness but my nights have taken on a new meaning of bittersweet. Thursday days are absolute beauty. I am feeling great, Ian goes to swimming class, Gina and I go to the gym, then we meet all the mommies out somewhere for the mommies to talk and the kids to play. It is really my favorite day of the week because without fail our Thursdays are awesome.

But as with all Thursdays, we all know what always comes next... Fridays! It has been this way for a long time, I guess since someone came up with the weekdays in a calendar. Meh, I really don't know those facts! These days Thursday nights mean the dread of the coming day, the wanting to curl up in a ball and say, "you can't make me go tomorrow" (if you were wondering I did used to do that to my mom when she would need to take me to the doctor). The knowing that my feeling great is short lived for the next few days....it is hard. I am ready to have my Thursday nights back to what they are meant for...one more day before the weekend.

Chemo chronicle 2.4 – May 7, 2011

I felt totally rushed in the morning and out of sorts and I was not sure why. My appointment wasn't until 9:45am, it was kind of odd. But I did use my Vitamix blender this morning and made a yummy smoothie with an apple, strawberries, blueberries, about 2 cups of spinach and chocolate protein powder...yummy delicious! After much running around making smoothies, packing Eric and me salads and getting all the stuff I wanted to work on together, we were off. Ian couldn't have been happier to be dropped off at Parker's house and Eric and I were off. We walked into an almost dark office. The power had gone out. Crazy! Dr. H came in and we talked about my upcoming scan. She is VERY optimistic of great results. I told her I already have my mind on it being ALL gone!!

I got into the infusion room with no big drama, counts were all great and good to go. I did have an extra bag of bone strengthener added today, so that added on a little more time. I worked on card packs that I was donating to my church, Eric worked on rigging his phone's Wi-Fi to his computer because theirs was down today eh, whatever. I am never really sure what he was doing! I knew I felt different as soon as I got home. I was really loopy and tired and stayed that way for the rest of the day. I was thinking the extra bag really took it out of me and now all I wanted was a big juicy hamburger. Just like when I was pregnant. My iron levels were the only ones that were low so bring on the meat! Eric went and got me one after Ian was down because Ian was not having any of this going out to eat business. Whatever, this was easier! After eating way too much, I passed out on the couch at 8:30pm. You would think it was 2:30 am, I was drunk, and just downed some Whataburger. Not the case!!

Wham bam – no thank you ma'am – May 8, 2011

This has hands down been the worst treatment to date. I would easily take a crappy infusion compared to this. I guess I can say today is better. I only feel like crap today. As opposed to yesterday when I felt like complete sh*t. This is not the norm, THANK YOU GOD. It is the bone medicine Zoledronic Acid that is used to help strengthen my bones. From what Eric read, this should be a one-time gig, again THANK YOU GOD. My bones hurt like nothing I have ever felt, even my ankles and toes hurt. My skin hurts, even when Ian hugs me it hurts. I am cold even outside in the heat. I am so tired but I can't sleep and I can't get up and do anything because when I stand I think I might throw up. I tried to go to the Ladies Tea yesterday at church but had to leave about half way through – I hurt too much. We went to church this morning and I was a wreck. I cried more than usual and I just couldn't get centered. I am praying that tomorrow this hurt is gone because my heart hurts too.

She taught me…. – May 9, 2011

She taught me that

even when I thought

I had nothing left to give,

that I had to dig a tiny bit deeper

 and I would find

I had a lot left to give.

She taught me that I made my bed

now I must lie in it

but I sure as hell can get out of that bed and re-make it.

She taught me friends are meant to be cherished...

especially with a bottle or two of wine!

She taught me to dream big

then go out there and make that dream come true.

She taught me how to step back,

look at the facts

not to panic,

and to do what needs to be done

in any situation.

She taught me life isn't always sweet as pie

but it is always worth living,

doing, being.

She taught me

how to be a mother myself.

I love you mom.

I know this is a day late but I feel this every day – not just on Mother's day. And hey, I'm usually a day or so late with my cards so this is quit fitting!!

Coming out of the fog... - May 10, 2011

Today is a new day!! I FINALLY feel like I have climbed out of the fog that I was stuck in for the past three days. Those were possibly the toughest three days I have had in a really long time. After talking to Eric last night I figured out that it took a huge emotional toll on me too. I went from feeling great, thinking this sh*t ain't so bad, from my off week...to being slammed head first into a brick wall. But, my fever broke last night (or I was having my first hot flash) and I woke up this morning feeling much, much better. Yesterday's daily word was just what I needed: RECOVERY!

I am healthy and whole and continually renewed by the spirit of God within me. Prayer is primary to my healing, whether I am recovering from an illness, surgery or even a broken heart. I begin each day with quiet moments of prayer. I give thanks for the life within me. I visualize the healthy, happy, energetic life I desire. Healing takes time, and recovery takes many forms. A positive outcome will result if I give my body and mind the time they need. Patiently, I pray for the wisdom to know and do all I can to facilitate my recovery. Turning my attention to the needs of others often helps my own recovery. Volunteering, even in a seemingly small way, renews me. Praying for others helps us all. Each prayer and every healthful activity supports my ongoing recovery.

I worked on thank you cards yesterday, necklace flowers and that made a world of difference in me, to me, and for me. It is too easy to get caught up in my own head about the hurt, the suck of it, the pissed off of me, but then something so simple as writing a thank you card totally changes me. I remember the love that person has for me and I for them and it gets me out of *that* place.

Lately, several people have been really worried about me. Don't be, I am better. I just needed to wallow in my own self-pity for a while; and no, this is NOT something I recommend, it didn't get me anywhere good.

Ian asked me to make him a date with his friends today and I already have it all organized and I am so excited to be getting out of the house with him to enjoy our day. Here's to being out of the fog.

33 – May 13, 2011

I like to look at my birthday every year how a lot of people look at New Year's. A new year with a clean slate for me to do with it what I wish. And I feel this year is no different. I can't say my 30's have rocked in the traditional way. I feel like my body has failed me but from body failure so much has happened and yes I am thankful that all this crap happened/is happening when I was in my 30s. I am pretty sure if it happened when I was 25 I would have had a major melt down, wouldn't have been able to see the silver lining and would have been drunk a lot more than I already was! And when I was 25 I didn't have Eric.

SO my goals for my 33rd year:

1. Au revoir cancer – FOREVER.

2. Start new postcard project (coming soon!!).

3. Take a kick a*s trip with Eric and Ian.

4. Take a romantic get away with Eric – who is up for watching Ian?!?!

5. AND – this is a scary one but with the help of a friend, I am going to put this blog into an e-book – there I said it!!! I am working on my fucking outline. I HATE OUTLINES! Don't worry, I will save some juicy stuff just for the book, I can't show all my cards on the blog! (And now you are reading it...BOOM! See what happens when you set goals!).

6. Maybe stop using so many curse words?? Maybe...probably not.

I don't really curse this much in "real" life – sometimes.

7. Continue to live life, enjoy it all, laugh, love, shine my light, help others, smile from my heart, see beauty in little things, and hug more. I really need to work on the hug more part!

8. Write in my journal daily (already do and want to keep up with it).

9. Meditate/pray at least 20 minutes daily (again, already do).

10. Get out and sell my necklaces to boutiques.

11. Send in my stuff to be considered as a designer for a scrapbook company. Why not? I need to scrapbook more and this would make me do it!

What have I learned thus far in life:

1. Finding love was 100% worth all the bullshit I went through with others. I grew from every relationship I had. I was just who I needed to be when I met Eric.

2. Tell people you love them....in person, on the phone, in a letter. I don't care just do it often. I just recently learned this, I would keep it to myself because I was scared they didn't love me back, but now I don't care. You don't have to love me back for me to love you...ask Ian, I still kiss on him all the time even though he tells me, "Mommy, you can't kiss me forever!" *Wanna bet???*

3. Listen to your heart. More than likely any question you have, your heart has already told you the answer. Now it might not be the answer you actually want to hear but it is THE answer. Your heart speaks very quietly but has the loudest message.

4. Being a stay at home mommy is hard but worth it all. It doesn't pay well in terms of money but that is easy to get over when

you get daily jokes, dances just to make me laugh, a few hugs and kisses, art work, laughter, songs, constant why's, a few balls thrown at your head, playing hide and seek and SO much more.

5. When someone repeatedly shows up in your life take notice. God has put them there for a reason. Gina and I constantly ran into each other, she claims she noticed me walking Ian while I was bald the first go around and thought to herself, she could be a friend. (Now of course I have to call bullshit, because I am sure was probably scared of catching what I had!) Anyway, God was trying to get us two together for some time before we let ourselves go into complete friendship and now, this train is rolling.

6. If you look around, your problems really aren't THAT bad. Someone always has it worse than you. And when you help others, your problems just seem to disappear.

7. Love is a powerful thing and can get us through a lot.

8. Not to take myself so seriously. This is a hard one but so important. I want to be perfect in what I do. I want such and such to be perfect but I am learning it doesn't really matter. Really, none of it matters. Taking time to listen to yourself/your heart, talk with God, love your family and friends, help others, look at the beauty in nature and all around us, now that's what matters.

9. Take it all one step at a time. I was listening to a Wayne Dyer cd the other day and he summed it up so nicely. When he sits down to write a book he doesn't look at the 300 hundred pages it needs to be. He looks at the chapters and focuses on one at a time. And trying not to smoke/drink/eat sugar, whatever, don't look at it for life look at it for today. Today I won't eat sugar, today I won't smoke/drink it is amazing what you can do for a day.

10. Holding on to the past of unforgiven stuff is like holding on to an old bag of nasty food. It doesn't hurt anyone but you. It doesn't stink up the other person's life and it takes up so much time and effort to hold it out from you so it doesn't touch you. Throw the

crap away already.

11. Count your blessing every day. Say thank you to God for all the wonderfulness you have in your life. So, here's to my 33rd birthday. I couldn't ask for more…family, friends, love, joy, laughter, heart, happiness…my cup does run over. Love to you.

Chemo Chronicle 2.5 – May 14, 2011

Ugh, I have been waking up around 5:00am every morning; wide awake, uncomfortable and not able to get back to sleep. My body is still very tired so I don't feel like getting up. I wish I did feel like getting up. Then I go back to sleep around 6:00am to 6:45am and without fail I have the weirdest dreams, just odd. Anyway, we were all up and rolling at 6:45am.

Eric and Ian had several sweet cards for me and Eric got me a new silver band since my wedding and engagement bands don't fit my chemo/steroid swollen finger. It made me sad not to be able to wear something, so he got me this simple band. I really love it!

At 8:10am we were out the door heading to Gina's to drop off Ian. Parker and Ian were like kids in a candy store when Ian got there. You would think they never saw each other, it is super sweet though. By 8:45 we are at my appointment. I didn't have to see anyone today, so it was straight to the infusion room for blood draw and treatment. My nurse who poked my port today was WONDERFUL!! And after she was done I told her, "Wow, you're great!" and you would have thought I just told her *You just won a million dollars!* She was so grateful for me to tell her that she was great at that. I can't imagine how beat down they get with people bitching and moaning all day. Why are you doing this, why am I still here, blah, blah, blah.

I actually didn't take anything with me to work on today because I needed some sleep. I knew if I had stuff to do I wouldn't sleep. I watched The Office, and then turned on Pandora and cat napped. At 11:00am I was done!! Busting out of this joint. It was funny, when I was getting "unhooked" a friend came over to chat and she turned her head away so as not to see what was happening on me. I feel the same way, I have no idea what the needle in my chest looks like being put in or out and am completely fine with that. We went to eat at Jorge's, a super yum Mexican food place that uses free range/grass feed meat! By 12:30pm I was home and in bed. Gina said she was fine having Ian until 2:30ish, so I decided I really needed to get some real rest. At 1:30ish I got a text from Josie telling me Gina ran over her phone. I had to laugh!! All in all this has been a great day. I already feel better than I did last Friday, so here is to hoping tomorrow is easy cheesy!

My birthday – May 15, 2011

All I can say is wow! Wow to what awesome friends I have. They threw me a hats and scarves party on Thursday night and it was just what I needed, yummy food, wine (maybe a little too much for me), cupcakes, great pictures of the evening and most importantly an abundance of wonderful friends. It really was a magical evening with the girls. After they sang happy birthday, I cried. I cried for me, for my wish to be cancer free forever, for my wonderful friends, for my broken heart being healed a little every day. I cried for all of it. I cried to cleanse and make room for the new.

I think there were more tears flowing than just mine so to add fuel to the fire; I decided it was a good time for me to read what I wrote:

You girls are my rocks,

my net of love,

my strength.

You girls each holds a piece of my heart

and each has helped paint my soul.

You girls make me laugh,

make me cry,

sometimes make me scream.

You girls

are my light when my road gets dark.

You girls

are the chorus to my song

and without it my song would be flat and boring.

You girls

are more than friends,

are more than I could ever have imagined in my life.

I love you girls.

This was to all the girls in my life, those who are here and those not able to be here. I loved every minute of the night. I loved the laughing, hugging, remembering, sharing of stories with new and old, enjoying the moment, the pure moment of the night. When Amanda left, she told me, "You look happy, really happy." She summed it up with those simple words. I am happy – happy to be where I am today, tomorrow and always.

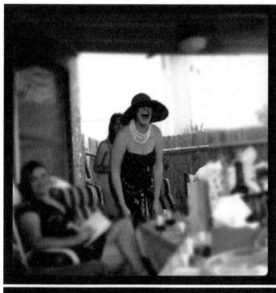

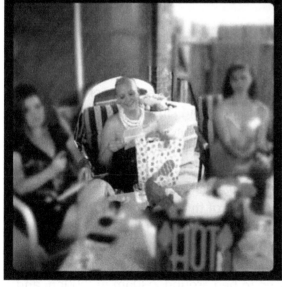

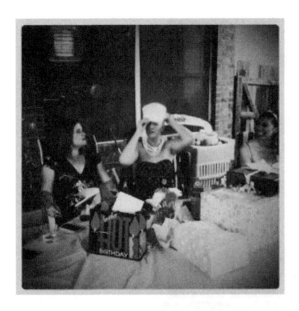

Chemo Chronicle 2.6 – May 20, 2011

I can't believe this was my 6th chemo. These treatments were
flying by. Fridays come and go now and I just keep track of the
number of treatments. I pretty much have the week down to a
science though which was really nice. Friday morning I feel great,
after treatment I am all kinds of loopy and tired, Friday night I have
to crash early. Saturday morning I wake up feeling great. It is really
odd. The feeling good lasts most of the day then Saturday night I
have to go down early. Sunday and Monday I feel blah, tired and
achy. It isn't anything too bad but I do get a little irritable with
people. I try not to, but that is what I do when I am tired. Ask Eric,
he will tell you! I usually go to bed around 7:30pm or 8:00pm and
sleep all through the night. Tuesday I wake up and can tell I turned
the corner. I feel good, not great yet but really good. I am able to
work out, play with Ian all day and hold up my end of the bargain
as a mommy. Wednesday and Thursday I am back to myself. My
energy is back, achiness is gone and I say bye-bye to the blahs. It

was really weird how it works but all in all, it isn't that bad. I am really looking forward to my scan on Wednesday!

I have a CT scan in about a week to see how this chemo is working. As always, I am asking for prayers.

Labels – May 23, 2011

I was listening to a CD the other day and on it they said, as soon as we put a label on someone we unknowingly and automatically put that something in a box. We all do it all the time. We label each other all day every day. That person isn't healthy because she doesn't eat the way I do. That person is not as spiritually advanced as me because she doesn't mediate the way I do. That person is not going to Heaven because he doesn't believe exactly what I do. That person is not successful because she doesn't have as big a house as me. Do you see how these labels can hold someone down, can change us if we are the ones being labeled? They can change us unknowingly. They can change us into believing this nonsense.

I realized the impact of labels when a friend of mine was talking to me about a friend of hers who has stage IV breast cancer. When she spoke of her friend to me, she would say, she has stage IV cancer also. It took me a minute to connect the dots of *also*. Who else has stage IV breast cancer? Oh, I guess I do. But the thing is I don't consider myself to have stage IV cancer. In fact I don't really even consider myself as having cancer. Yes, maybe in my medical chart I am "labeled" as this but in my heart, in my mind, in my life I don't. I can't put this label on myself or on others. The only time I have even thought of myself of stage IV was the day I was told this and I was handed a nice little brochure of what it means. I handed that brochure to Marci and Gina when we got home from that appointment and never again have I thought of myself as "that."

Do others label me as "cancer"? Is that all others see me as now? I feel like as soon as I allow people to label me as stage IV cancer, I am in a box. Stuck there with nothing else to do/to be but to have cancer. I am so much more than cancer. I am a wife, a mom, a daughter, a sister, a friend, an artist, a lover, a sharer of life, an encourager and so much more. I don't want to be in a box. I am much too restless to stay put in a box.

Drum roll please - May 26, 2011

So I just got a call from my Dr. H's office with my scan results.

It was at 1:40pm this afternoon. I had my phone with me all morning, willing it to ring. Then when I was done thinking about it and trying to get us out of the mall and home... it rang

I about hit the ceiling when it rang. Like I hadn't been waiting for it all morning! The only other time I waited for a call like this was when I was waiting to hear from the breast surgeon for my results the first time. We stopped in the middle of JC Penny. Tammy and I were both holding our breath.

You curious at all??

EXCELLENT!!!! Is what the nurse said as soon as she told me who was calling! She said it was written all over my chart. *HELL YES* it is written all over my chart!!!

I yelled, I danced and then Tammy and I cried. SO, here is what I "heard"....we will know 100% what is going on next Friday. What is GONE: the big ass spot in the middle of my lungs that was around my lymph nodes and all but TWO little spots in my lungs. The two that are still there, one in lower left is tiny and one spot in lower right. Both spots are "dense" and that doesn't necessarily mean cancer. They don't know about the bone spots because those didn't show up on the CT only on the PET scan. What there is NOT: any new uptake, which is GREAT! That means no new cancer!!!!

I asked if I still need chemo. She said she wasn't sure but to keep all appointments as is for now. Here is what I am thinking, you know since I am so well versed in oncology, that I will get two more months of chemo (F*IN BREEZE!!). That will be followed by a PET scan, which will show I am ALL clear. I will then wipe my hands of this mess and Eric and I will get on with our lives!!!!!! BUT that was just my thinking. I am not even sure I have processed this yet. I know I haven't. I still feel shaky and in a fog of WHAT IN THE WORLD is happening, but I am SO SO SO thankful for my answered prayers. Everyone's answered prayers. I knew my prayer of "Thank You sweet Father for the miracle of my cancer free body today, tomorrow and always" was working. I knew it in my heart. I knew it in my soul. Thank you all for your prayers, your love, and your support. I know this isn't over yet, but I am a hell of a lot closer to the finish line than 2 months ago. I am still dumbstruck so if this doesn't make sense please forgive me.

A Healed Heart – May 27, 2011

A heart can break,

A heart can heal,

It will heal.

Though the healing process

Puts the heart back together,

The heart can never be put back together

Exactly the way it was before it broke.

Some pieces might be left out,

Some pieces will be arranged differently,

Some new pieces will be added.

A heart can break;

A heart can heal,

No matter what a healed heart changes people.

This is another one I wrote sometime last year. I had just been put on my anti-depressant after treatment and was starting to feel "normal" again but I noticed that me, my normal, my "everything" was different. Not a bad different – just different from before...but why wouldn't I be different? I grew, I healed, I conquered. I can't wait to see how this broken heart heals.

Project Sending Love – May 31, 2011

This is it. This is the big project I have been "talking" about when I kept saying I had something in the works. I 100% feel this is one of my big to-dos in this life. I believe God has tasked me with this to help others and I send love out into the world, one person at a time. This idea has been in my head since the start of my diagnosis the first time. It has evolved through many stages, it has been pushed to the back burner and completely off the stove several times, but it just wouldn't go away. My heart always held a piece of this idea no matter what I tried to do instead.

What is Sending Love? It is simple; it is a way for me, you, and everyone to write thoughts, feelings, kind word, and love for others down and send it to them. From the ProjectSendingLove blog: After both diagnoses, I received the most heartfelt cards from friends and family. These cards were filled with words of love, kindness, joy, hope and prayers. I honestly think this love helped carry me through cancer with flying colors! Why do we wait to tell each other how much we love one another, how important someone is to us and what an impact the person makes on our lives and the world until a tragedy strikes? What if we all started sharing the love, kindness, joy and prayers that we think about others in our hearts all the time with those we are thinking about? How special and important would they feel? How could that love for each other change the world? I am not sure, but I have to see.

It is easy to get caught up in the idea of "how" I tell others that I love them, respect them, that they are very important to me, to the world. But the how is the easiest part, open your heart and love. You can't run out of it and the more you give, the more you have to give and the more you get. Crazy little thing God gave us, the ability to love. Sending Love is such a simple idea and even simpler to do: write your love for others down on a postcard and send it. I am tired of talking all this talk, now it is time for me to walk the walk.

"Be the change you want to see in the world." - Gandhi

Chemo Chronicle 2.7 – June 4, 2011

I didn't know what to expect going into this appointment being as I just had a CT scan. Would she tell me no more chemo like my friend heard a few weeks ago? Would she tell me we were going to change my schedule? Do less or more chemo? I just didn't know. The getting there was much easier this morning since Ian stayed home with my Aunt versus us taking him to Gina's, hence we didn't have to get him dressed and put together either. I might just have to start sending him to Gina's in pajamas.

The nurse doing my port was quite the character and really had me wondering if I should be letting this guy stick me in the chest. Seriously! He told me he "calms" people down by feeding them all this bullshit, then POKE and all is done. Well it worked because I was NOT thinking about the port poke with him telling us these stories. When Dr. H walked in she said, "There's my girl with the great scans" and gave me a big hug. That made it all real. I did have great scans. They didn't accidently call the wrong person. Until I heard it from her I didn't really want to believe it. She did say she was unexpectedly surprised by how well the first two rounds of chemo worked and that honestly she had never seen two rounds of Abraxane work that well. I told her I was an overachiever! And what I thought about me having two spots left on my lungs, I only have ONE TINY SPOT left. We still don't know about the bones but will in eight weeks! And yes, for those wondering...my oncology skills are spot on!

Two more rounds of chemo (so six more treatments) then a PET scan. I told her that is what I said she would say and we decided I might not need an oncologist anymore!! A few things I didn't know or think about. I didn't know HOW many spots in my lungs I started out with, but she told me it was around 20. I also didn't know how big "the big one" in the middle of my lungs was. Oh, it was about as big as a racquetball. There is a reason I don't ask certain questions.

I hadn't thought about my "maintenance" after I was done with chemo. I thought when I am done, I am done! That however is not the case. And the thing is they don't really have a maintenance protocol in place for triple negative people. Trip neg cancer isn't caused by something producing too much of something. She wants to talk with the MD Anderson doctor to see if they have or will be having any maintenance trials happening soon and if not, I might stay on abraxane once a month/every six weeks until something new comes out.

The good news is triple negative is the *hot topic* in cancer research right now, so hopefully there will be a maintenance drug out in the next two years that isn't chemo. I was a little in shock about all this yesterday. I just didn't think about having stuff to do after this chemo. I just so wanted to hear, 2 more rounds of this chemo and then done, done, DONE! This is not the case at all. I was talking to my friend who got clean scans after 6 months of chemo and it was nice to talk to her about this. We both agreed it is hard to be excited. Yes, it is an absolute miracle but it isn't over. It more than likely will never be over. It never occurred to me that I will be in some sort of treatment forever. That is what stage IV, or Metastatic Breast Cancer is; there is no stage five.

Continuing on – June 6, 2011

I received an email from a dear friend on Saturday titled, "Continuing on", after she read my chemo post and the news about my "done" not ever really happening. It took a bit for everything to really sink in, as it usually does with me. I needed some time to process it all, sort it out and get my feelings in order.

That is why I have never liked fighting in the heat of the moment, I don't have my argument together!

She wrote to me, "I am not trying to find a reason or lessen the impact, but the thought that came to me is that this will keep you in the zone. Too many times we stay centered in Spirit when we are in crisis and have every great intention of keeping up with our meditation and prayer when it is over, but then life gets hectic and we go back to our human lives..."

And the funny thing is, I have thought this before. I have thought what if I got cancer this second time to make me write again... really write from my heart, about my spirituality, about life, the good, the bad and the ugly. I sure didn't write from my heart after I was "cured" of cancer the first time.

Against the stream... – June 9, 2011

"What you choose to dedicate your time to matters not just for you but for all those who are affected by the withholding or the deliverance of your unique gifts. What are you dedicating your time to?" – Debbie Ford

I get these daily *life lessons* or whatever you want to call them. I love them. I love reading these little tidbits every morning with my cup of coffee. Yes, I still drink a cup of coffee every morning and I read my computer instead of a newspaper. I don't even go to real news sites; I really don't like the news. Back to the quote above, it was funny; this came when my hubby was deciding to change jobs. He had a very "cush" job where he was, but his heart wasn't in it anymore. He didn't feel he was using all his talents to better himself. He took a big step and changed jobs. He got lots of "whys" from others who are still at the old job. In terms of why leave a gravy train, why leave something you know, why leave "this"? But the thing is, "this" was filled with negativity. People always talking about what was wrong, what they weren't getting, blah, blah, blah. He left lots of stock options but in the end, those stock options, that money would never change the fact that he needed and craved something new, something better, something his heart was calling him to do. He stepped out, got a fresh breath of air and took a leap of faith, and I couldn't be more proud of him. He decided to swim against the stream instead of flowing with it. Going with the stream would have been easy but it wasn't getting him where he needs to be. It is hard to swim against the stream. It is hard to leave something you know for something you have no idea about. It is hard to take a deep breath, tell yourself you can and let go of that security blanket and walk away.

It is hard. But it is oh so worth it. Believe me, I am preaching from experience here. I held so tight to that security blanket I quit my job before my first round of breast cancer. I knew my job, I was good at it, but it didn't give my spirit a boost, it didn't make my heart sing. It didn't do much of anything besides give me a paycheck and guilt that I wasn't home with Ian. I was scared though. I was scared of what life would be without that paycheck. I now look back at the craziness of that. Yes at first it was a little tough to know I wasn't "contributing" to our bank accounts, but then I realized I was contributing to life, Ian's spirit and heart, and to us, our family. Once I stepped out of the "norm" and looked at us, our lives, what I/we needed, there was no choice to be made, my heart had spoken and it was time for me to swim against the stream. I am not saying what I did is what all people want. But I am saying if your heart is telling you that something needs to change, that something isn't right. Listen. You don't have to do something

about it right now but listen. Your heart knows the way and it is
has an amazing story to tell if we will listen.

Chemo Chronicle 2.8 – June 11, 2011

First of all, it completely freaks me out that I have already had
8 rounds of chemo. Last time 8 was my magic number. I had 8
rounds total and I was done or so I thought.

Today was an easy day in terms of chemo. My appointment was at
8:15am, so it was up and at 'em early around here today. Gina told
me that we could bring Ian over in his pajamas today, and he was
beyond thrilled about that! It was hard in terms of realizations. I
was extremely tired. I was not sure if I was just wearing down or if
it was the fact it was hotter than hell outside. We went to a small
water park Thursday and for some crazy reason Ian didn't nap. I
ended up going to bed at 7:30pm Thursday night and slept ALL
night. Yes, I slept 11 hours. I asked the nurse when she brought
me the sheet with my blood count read outs on it if my red count
being a little low was the reason I was so tired. She kind of laughed
and said my red blood count wasn't really "that" low and I was
going through a little thing called chemo. And she nailed it when
she said, "And I bet you don't slow down. You just added this to
your to-do list" and she was right.

Up until about 2 weeks ago I was going all out. I did everything I
had been doing but I broke a few weeks ago, and I broke hard. Like
my whole egg cracked and my yolk was running out everywhere. I
realized I couldn't do it all anymore and when I was totally honest
with myself, I realized I didn't want to do it all. Yes, I was the only
one expecting me to do it all. I still wanted to be super woman but
I now know I have to say no. I have to say no to what doesn't help
me heal, what doesn't help me rest, what doesn't help me be the

best mom, wife, me I can be. I have to say no. Saying no is hard for me. I want to do everything I am invited to do. I want to be there for my friends as they are here for me. I want to; but, the reality of my life right as that I can't. Not how I used to be able to be there.

Like me and my life as it changes, my relationships have to change also. My family, my health and spirituality are the most important things to me right now and always. So if I have to miss get-togethers, lunch dates, play dates, taking orders for Leopards & Lilies and many other things, I need to, I have to, I will. Just when I think I have it all figured it out, life dictates a new role for me.

OUT OF CONTROL!!! – June 15, 2011

I feel 100% out of control in my life right now, in so many areas I don't even know where to start. Out of control with my body and what it is doing. I "thought" I had my after chemo schedule down but these past few weeks nothing is the same as it was. I am thoroughly exhausted all the time, I have a dull ache most of the week and my stomach is doing some weird things.

Out of control with the house, now don't get me wrong, I have never been one to really keep the house all that picked up, but this is something that is adding to my lack of control; a messy house, but I don't have the energy to pick it up daily.

Out of control with my emotions, I feel I am short with people, I feel like I snap at nothing with Ian, I feel like I never know what is around the next corner. And what sucks even more is the more I feel out of control, the more I try to control something and being as I am with Ian most days this leads to me trying to control his actions, which is the silliest thing ever trying to control a 3 year olds actions. The actions I am trying to control aren't even important in the grand scheme of things. I just want to be in control of something. And I find myself looking at me through his eyes and wondering what happened to his mommy who was healthy, active and easy going but is now a ball of stress because I feel like everything else is crumbling around me. I have to take a step back and ask myself if this really matters and the answer is most always no, it just sucks that I have to do it so many times a day.

A fine line – June 22, 2011

A fine line between too much and not enough

A fine line between care about me, care for me, and leave me the hell alone

A fine line between asking how I am and ignoring the fact I go to chemo 3 out of 4 weeks

A fine line between my smiles and my tears

A fine line I walk everyday

A fine line that sometimes I am on both sides at once

Neither side is better; neither side is easier, neither side is safer

A fine line of feeling good of feeling like shit

A fine line of living in limbo not knowing what tomorrow will bring

A fine line that can blur all too easily

I actually wrote this back in March, right after I started chemo...I still feel this way most days...It is hard to walk to the line...

Yes... - June 24, 2011

Yes I am ok, well, getting there

Yes I started back on my "happy pills"

Yes my body is one big unbalanced mess

Yes I am starting to work out again

Yes the help you send/give is MUCH appreciated

Yes I am so ready to get my PET scan

Yes I believe in my heart that all the cancer is gone

Yes I still leave it all in God's hands

Yes my face is crazy dry

Yes I have neuropathy in my left thumb and index fingers

Yes my other nail beds feel like I smashed them in a door

Yes I still remember to laugh – really a lot of the time

Yes I love on Ian daily

Yes it warms my heart

Yes I thank God daily for Eric

Yes he is my strength

Yes I let Ian watch too much tv

Yes I am ok with it – for now

Yes I am creating again

Yes it helps me heal

Yes I will continue to talk about my grief

Yes I know it helps

Yes I promise to not pretend all is well when it is bad

Yes I know my normal has changed

Yes I am starting to accept it

Yes I promise – I will be okay

Yes I am sure

It's Back…- June 27, 2011

My creativity, my desire to create, my interest in creating and my knowing how much creating helps me, helps me heal from the inside out. I am not sure if it is the fact that Jill came and helped me clean/organize my craft room or if it's because I started taking Lexapro again. Maybe it's because I have made a VERY conscious effort to pull myself out of this slump, talk about it and lean on God, family, and friends more. Whatever the case, I am feeling so much better knowing just knowing that I am feeling better. Does that make sense? Anyhow, I made this canvas for Ian's room.

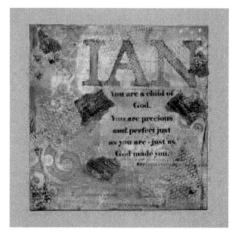

I want him to know in his heart that God loves him, that he is precious and perfect in God's eyes no matter what. I want him to know this, to hear it on a daily basis and I figured it hanging on his wall for us to read to him daily is a great way to ingrain it in him. I am really enjoying painting again, it does help me heal.

Chemo Chronicle 2.10…- July 2, 2011

I really can't believe I am starting my 4th cycle. On one hand it seems like these past 3 cycles have all gone so fast but on the other hand, I feel like we have been dealing with this forever. Time is such a funny thing. After dropping a very excited Ian off to a very excited Parker, we were off. Just knowing how much they love each other and what a great time Ian has over there makes it SO much easier to leave him for a few hours. We had a great visit with Dr. H, and yes, that is what we do, we talk and laugh about stuff going on in our lives. We don't just talk about cancer and treatment.

We did figure out the name of the doctor I had seen at MD Anderson, which we were previously calling "the funny man" because none of us could remember his name and because he is pretty quirky. She needs to chat with him about my maintenance plan. Laurie and I decided that the word maintenance makes it sound like I am a car with a maintenance schedule to keep. Hey, if I can be a fine tuned, well running machine I will take it! We talked to Dr. H about my upcoming PET scan which she said was really looking forward to seeing the results, score one for Team S. I mean really, to hear her say that she is looking forward to the results as she expects to see negative…NEGATIVE CANCER really hit home with me. She believes as much as I do that this is gone! She didn't yell that at us, but she could have and I wouldn't have minded it at all! Also, she told us we can go ahead and plan a little vacation that following week, in my mind that means my current chemo schedule will not continue! So PET scan is on July 22nd and follow up with Dr H is on July 29th. I mean really, I cannot wait for that appointment! Other than that, same ole same ole: I got zometa for my bones; I feel ok this morning; I am tired but nothing too new on that front. My mom is taking Ian to a small water park today so Eric can get some work done around here and I can rest. Rest is good for me at this point in time!

Peace or Drama? – July 6, 2011

Do you want to be right or be happy? Do you want peace or drama?

These were two questions that our minister talked about one Sunday that really, really hit home with me.

You can't have both at the same time. You can't have peace and drama at the same time within yourself.

You can't want to be right and be happy at the same time.

One of them takes ego and the other takes heart/Spirit/love. I feel like a few weeks ago were filled with drama within myself, I wasn't allowing the peace to be in me. I wasn't allowing myself to get in that place that I know and love in my heart. I was only allowing myself to have turmoil within my heart and it was a bad feeling.

I was taking the simplest things to heart, thinking if someone said something it was automatically directed at me and my guard and defenses went up. Of course, I talked to Eric about it but his answers weren't what I was looking for. I wanted him to justify the fact that I **should** have my defenses up and possibly start an argument with these people. Then my next stop as always was

Marci, but when she told me the same thing I knew the drama was within me not with these other people. I had been down, feeling hopeless and like I was drowning. Once I made the decision that I was going to ask for help, get back on Lexapro, something in me changed, even before I started the medicine. I realized even though I needed a little extra help with medicine that it was still up to me to change my attitude and my thoughts, because the more I thought about feeling bad, the worse I felt. It took a lot of going inside my heart, praying for guidance and understanding with this and a lot not to get upset, not to let the negative thoughts get me down and keep me down and more importantly to just let go. For this I am thankful, I can tell I have grown and am continuing to grow into the person I want to be. One who forgives easily (yes, even myself), one who turns to God for strength and guidance and one who is happy, truly happy.

Chemo Chronicle 2.11 – July 9, 2011

Eleven….eleven chemos done.

This is all still so bizarre to me.

I sometimes wonder if this will ever really seem normal or will it always be bizarre to me, especially when I start maintenance? I am guessing it will always seem bizarre to me, just what is happening in my body, what the medicine is doing in there, what my body is capable of and is doing…it is a true miracle. I am definitely feeling that this was number 11.

I haven't been bouncing back near as fast as I was…who am I kidding, I am not bouncing back at all! I am pretty much either tired or exhausted all the time, even on Wednesdays and Thursdays which both used to be my "good" days.

Eh, so be it.

I still have to think that if tired is the worst of it, I can easily take it! I still have random bone pain but nothing is consistent from day to day. On one hand I wish it were so I could plan my days but on the other hand the bone pain not being consistent means sometimes I have it and sometimes I don't. See? All very bizarre!

Treatment this time was easy cheesy. I didn't have to see Dr. H or a nurse being as this was #2 of this round. At the end of my treatment though, I was talking to my infusion nurse about how zometa (bone medicine from last week) wipes me out. The man next to me overheard and suggested I get unflavored pedialyte. I never knew they had unflavored but like me, he doesn't eat sugar, hence the unflavored. It kind of tasted like watered-down pickle juice. It has a very odd after taste. Anyway, he told me he gets zometa once a month and until he figured out to do the pedialyte he was like me, exhausted. Then he tried the pedialyte and the hydration from it helped him feel good even after treatment. We also chatted a bit about diet. I love talking to people who take the same approach as us to this. It does help me know we aren't too crazy! He was given 12 months to live, 28 months ago! He cut all sugar, processed food, does mind/body/spirit approach as well! Really, this helped me SO much hearing this. It is hard to say no to wine, to eating out, to food at parties, but to know, really know that it made/will continue to make such a difference to my health, my no more cancer, makes it totally worth it.

Unknown – July 13, 2011

It hit me the other morning that I am scared of this coming Friday, scared of the unknown of what is to come next. It is almost 99% certain that this will be my last full round of chemo and that scares me and it scares me if this is NOT my last full round. I had a complete pathological response last time I had chemo, that means the chemo ate away all the cancer last time too. It scares me that it came back, it scares me to think about chemo again, it scares me to think about it coming back again. It all scares me.

There are a few facts that Eric and Gina like to keep pointing out to me. Really? One would think they get together and plan their defense speeches to me and all my arguments to them because their speeches are always the exact same, kind of annoying! I will be on maintenance this time and will have MANY more scans while on maintenance. I know this - I do, but the thought of going off full chemo does scare me. I have taken charge of my health this time around. Last time, I talked a good game but never really made huge changes. I figured, it was gone and that was that. The fact that I have cut sugar and processed foods out makes a huge difference. I don't really have other statistics to look at here. There really aren't many other women with trip negative metastatic who make it to maintenance, so yes this is a great achievement and a great stat to add for others in my situation. I DO know all this stuff...but it doesn't change the fact that I am scared of the unknown, of what is to come...I wish it did, but it just doesn't.

Chemo Chronicle 2.12 – July 17, 2011

12...12 chemos...way too many. When I look at this, it really doesn't surprise me how flippin' beat down tired I am. Nothing I do seems to help this tiredness. I can't sleep all day because, well that isn't natural, but I can't get up and actually do anything because I feel like I might just fall asleep at any given moment. My appointment on Friday was nothing exciting. My white blood count is down, so I need to be careful this week and next with germs. I am on edge about this coming Friday's PET scan. The nurse practitioner did tell me that I am "allowed" to call at 3:01 on Monday if I by chance I haven't heard from them. We were laughing because I told her I needed a time I was allowed to start calling and not seem like a crazy person pushing redial nonstop, so she said 3:01 is completely acceptable! I keep telling myself this is my last Sunday to feel this tired and this beat down...here's hoping!

A big, fat tantrum – July 21, 2011

Is what I want to throw, if I were an irrational 2 year-old. I kind of know why kids throw massive tantrums when their world is out of control, that out of control feeling sucks and sometimes they just need to voice their opinion of suckage. I was talking to Marci after a pretty rough day a few days ago and instead of calling her when I started feeling out of control I waited until I was full on out of control, which is fine with her because at least we can laugh at some of the sh*t that comes out of my mouth and yes, I am one of those that once I say something out loud it frees me of the thought that circulate through my mind. I figured out that this point in my life is so hard for me right now because all the coping mechanisms I have used for so long are no longer available in my bags of tricks.

Drinking alcohol, yes I admit it, I used alcohol to numb me to the situation, to celebrate something, to free me for as long as I can remember. Things weren't going so good? Go out for a drink. Wanted something fun to do? Go out for a drink; just hang out with friends and drink. Broke up with a boyfriend? All the girls come drink. Rough day? A glass of wine at night...oh, who am I kidding, maybe a bottle!

Food, food has always been an emotional crutch for me since

as long as I can remember. Sad? Eat. Happy? Eat. Bored? Eat. Mad? Eat. Stressed? Eat. And what I would reach for was always carbs and sugar loaded food. Yes they made me feel better in the moment, but always left me wondering why I did that.

Exercise, I have been knocked back to walking and yoga. I feel like I have been asked to go to the back of line because I can't hang with the big girls. I will admit I haven't given either of these the real benefit of the doubt because I am still being a baby and throwing a fit about my lack of physical conditioning. But exercise, a good hard sweat used to clear my mind and get me centered and now, well let's just say the thought of me running more than 2 minutes makes me want to curl up and go to bed. I am trying to find new coping mechanisms to help me deal with this, with everyday stress, with life as I now know it.

Well....sh*t...the good, the bad and the in between – July 27, 2011

This is not at all what I had prepared myself for. I got the call late Monday afternoon with my PET scan results.

I am still numb, confused, pissed off and asking why?

What I thought was extremely good news now turns out to be just okay news.

I thought ALL the bone stuff was gone, but after getting the actual report yesterday and reading it, I still have stuff on my left shoulder. I so wanted all the bone stuff to be gone.

The bad news, the one spot on my lungs that was left has grown from 1.8 cm x 1.3 cm at the time of the CT in May to 2.4 cm x 1.4

cm now, and I think this is actually a lymph node, but I won't know for sure until Friday. And there is a new spot that is 4 mm...not big enough for the PET to tell what it is.

I am numb, I am not sure what to think, what to do, anything. This seems to be a bigger shock to me than the diagnoses, but I may have just forgotten that already. From what Eric has read, this isn't all that uncommon. It was uncommon how well I responded to the Axbraxian in the first place. He also read that many people have to try a few different chemos through their journey because the cancer adapts to the chemo, which is just so crazy to me. I was just so sure I was done. I was so sure everything was working the way it should....I was so sure of it all. I just wanted a break from this so badly. I just didn't want to have to think about "what ifs" anymore. I feel defeated. But not for a second will I stop fighting...

I have too much to fight for - July 30, 2011

I guess it is time I write this. I was thinking if I didn't write it or talk about it that it would somehow not be true and go away. I am pretty sure that is not actually the case. Yesterday was a really, really hard day.

Here are the facts, I am not sure how so much got lost in translation from the CT report in May to now. I think we were all on such a high from the great response, Eric and I didn't ask enough questions.

The spot that was a huge cluster on the front of my lungs was the spot that was left after the CT scan. I was under the impression that whole thing was gone, not so much. That is the spot that has grown since the May CT scan. We can't just have it removed surgically because it is all twisted up in blood vessels and what not. There is a new spot but too small to show actual uptake. The spot on my left shoulder is still there it hasn't gotten bigger or smaller and there is still some on my right rib.

I am so grateful that we knew about most of this on Monday otherwise yesterday would have been a complete mess. We had time to digest the news and get our questions together before actually talking to Dr. H.

So I started on a new chemo cocktail yesterday: carboplatin and gemcitabine. We are also trying to get me into a trial for Iniparib. I should know about this next week.

These two chemos are more intense than what I was on with more potential for side effects. However, with this combo and the parp inhib (trial stuff) they have had great response. I am going to start asking y'all for specific prayers. I have heard people having true miracles happen from this. My prayer for this week is: to get into the trial and not feel side-effects. Eric and I allowed ourselves to have our pity party last night and get it all out on the table, but today we woke up fresh and ready to take it on. We are well aware I more than likely will be in chemo for quite some time, but peace has been made with that fact. I was questioning how long I can go on like this, but after today doing what we do; I know I can do this forever. I might just need to sleep more than normal people.

Chemo Chronicle 3.2 – August 6, 2011

I still haven't heard anything on the trial. The research nurse is 99% confident I will get in, but says she won't be happy until we have it in writing. I am going with that also. Treatment was easier today. It lasted a little over 3 hours and instead of watching trashy TV I decided to meditate and envision my cancer cells being blown up by the chemo. Hey, whatever I can do to help. My white blood count is low, so I have to get a Nuelasta shot on Monday. Oh joy! (Read in your most sarcastic voice.) Last week's treatment treated me pretty good. I was really tired, but I never got too nauseated. I just felt morning sickness a few days but nothing that made it impossible to go on with the day. I did have trouble eating which sucks. Nothing but crap sounds good, so on one hand this is affecting me a lot like A/C did (the first chemo I ever did). I think all this is catching up with Ian which seriously breaks my heart. He told Gina last week that he didn't like going to her house because it always meant I had to go to the doctor. She is so great with him and told him that no matter if he was at her house or home with BB, I would still have to go to the doctors. Both Eric and I have made a conscience effort to talk as openly as possible with him about it, which is so hard. I want to shelter him from all this, but that is not looking like it is possible. I made him an appointment for Wonders & Worries in two weeks. We hadn't done this before because well, we didn't think this was going to go on for this long. Now, well, we don't know when it will actually end.

It seems that people did like the specific prayer requests from last week, so I am going to continue those. Please pray that I get into the trial and that my energy returns for Ian's birthday party next Saturday. We are keeping it small this year because in the past he was overwhelmed with the amount of people who were there. Eric read somewhere a kid should have the number of guests at the party as the age they are turning. We aren't doing only four guests but maybe a few more than that. He got to make his guest list of his friends and I just said ok, it is your party you invite your friends! I really hope this party lives up to his expectations. He has been talking about it since March.

Pictures, trials, birthdays – oh my! – August 10, 2011

Pictures: My neighbor Holly, who is a photographer, took some pictures of me back in June. She posted them on her blog and I am honestly still in awe of the sweet comments from her blog followers. I have never thought of myself as "stunning" as she likes to tell me people are posting on her blog, so it has taken me a while to post them here. It is one thing on her blog. I mean she did take the pictures but on my blog, I don't know. It is always scary posting pictures of yourself...you know? Then she told me today that she entered a black and white contest and it was picked from thousands of other pictures, which completely blows me away. Anyway, I must admit as one, who really doesn't like to be the center of attention, it feels awesome for her to send me all the amazing comments from this picture too.

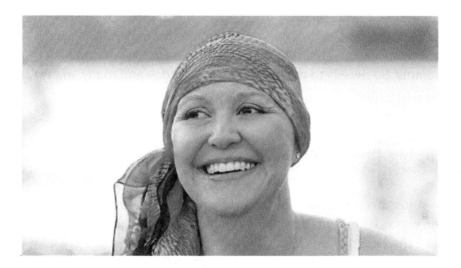

Trials: YIPPIE, I got word today that I was accepted for the parp trial!! This is great news. Eric has been asking my doctor about parps from the get go. He told me he really feels this is the right path for me. I will go with him on that thought being as he is the one out of us two who does the research! This does mean though, that I will be getting infusions on Fridays AND Mondays which is a huge pain in my ass. But hey if it works, I will get infusions two days a week forever if I need to. I will be on a two week on/one week off schedule now. I am off this Friday and will start all the parp next Friday.

Ian's 4th birthday is tomorrow. A big shift has happened in me these last few months. Before all this cancer nonsense, I was dreading Ian growing up. I wanted him to stay my baby forever. Now I am so excited about his birthday tomorrow and all others to come. I now just want to see him grow up. It is that plain and simple. I also realize that life goes on no matter how much we try to stop it or how much we wish things were different. Life goes on, day by day. I have had a rough couple of months not feeling good, wondering if I was possibly driving myself crazy (that is still up for debate), feeling like I am continually going through the grieving cycle, but looking at him reminds me I am here today to be his mommy. So here is to my big boy's 4th birthday and many, many more to come.

The big 4!! – August 14, 2011

Well, just like Christmas, birthdays come and go superfast. This one was no different, but I am VERY happy to say that it lived up to all the expectations Ian had for it. He told both me and Eric that this was the best birthday ever. I am not really sure he remembers the others, but it made my heart smile. We had a great birthday weekend. My mom, sister and nephews were here to help Ian celebrate and he couldn't have been happier. Now we are in the midst of a toy cleanout. Man alive, how do we have so many toys? I have also started writing Ian letters. This is the one I wrote him for his birthday:

Dear Ian,

Wow! I really can't believe that you are 4 years old today. You amaze me daily with your loving heart, sweet nature and ability to make me laugh! You become more empathic daily being concerned with other's feelings and wellbeing. If someone is hurt or needs help, you are the first to run and tell me. You play really well with your friends with the occasional *fight*. I have tried to tell you if someone hits or pushes you first that it is okay to hit/push back to stick up for yourself, but you aren't big on this. You aren't a fighter in one little bit. You are a lover and want everyone to be peaceful and just get along. You always know just what to do to make me laugh, even if you are getting in trouble, which is really not very often at all. You have this dance you do that no matter what is happening will make me laugh out loud. You often do this dance just to make me laugh. I can tell making me laugh is one of your priorities and I must admit that I do love it.

You already have a little engineer's mind. You want to know how everything works and sometimes I have to tell you that you need to ask daddy because I honestly don't know how it all works. You love to play games and hate to lose. I try to explain winning isn't everything, but you don't want to hear it. You don't really like to play by yourself yet, so we play together most of the time when we are at home. You love daddy telling you stories at night, anyone reading you books, chocolate milk, grape juice, apples slices, talking all the time and so much more. I can say this summer you officially learned to swim on your own! You even jump off the diving board by yourself. Of course daddy was the first one of us to let you do it because even though I knew you could, it made me nervous. You are the light of my life and I love you with all my heart. I can't wait to see you grow up my little man.

Love,

Mommy

Acceptance... - August 17, 2011

We booked a trip to Michigan for my next off week. We had been holding off booking any trips until "this" was all over, but I think we are now accepting the fact that "this" might never really be over; that I could possibly be on some sort of chemo for a very long time, even forever. That is not an easy thing to accept by any means. I am still trying to accept that Ian will one day have to learn to accept his mommy has cancer and our life will inevitably be much different than the lives of his friends. I have accepted that wine is no longer in my bag of tricks and food is now for fuel and not for an emotional crutch. I am still trying to accept that I might possibly be bald for the rest of my life. I am learning to accept emotional support from others and not try to be so strong all the time. I have been doing better and if I feel like crying to whomever, I cry. I don't try to hold it back. I even let Gina hug me while I was crying the other day at swim school. Now that is emotional progress for me!

I have accepted our family of three is perfect just the way it is; accepting that this life is now my life, our life has not been easy. I had been in denial for many months, I admit it. I kept thinking that the four months of my first chemo was going to be it, I could wash my hands of this again and go on. I am truly now accepting *that* scenario, as awesome as it would have been, is not the case. And will never be the case.

Chemo Chronicle 3.3 – August 21, 2011

It was a hard day. I admit it, I don't do well with change....AT ALL!
I like to know what is going to happen, where I am going, what
it looks like, etc. Yes, Ian is just like me in regards to this. I felt a
little like a lost 4 year old Friday when we walked into the office
in Round Rock. My doctor moved offices to a new location and
today was the first day there. I am still not sure about it all as with
most new things. It is a lot smaller but it is oddly too small. I know,
weird. The infusion room is a lot louder due to the smaller size and
it doesn't seem things here are as streamlined as they were at the
old office. Eric keeps telling me that this is just as new to them as it
is to me, which is true.

They had to hire a whole slew of people to come over to this office
since they just made it bigger. That was just the start of the hard
day. With my new infusion of BSI (trial drug) it adds another hour
onto the infusion. So now a normal Friday infusion will be at least
3.5 hours and when I have to get Zometa (bone stuff) it will be
around a four and half to five hour day. We checked in at 8:15am
to see my doctor and didn't leave until 2:00pm and it wasn't even
a Zometa day. The whole time I was sitting in the infusion chair all I
could think about was how in the world are we going to make this
work with Ian's school? His school will be from 9:30am – 2:30pm.
There is no way I can drop him off and pick him up on Fridays. Yes
Eric can do one/both of them, but how long is his work going to be
cool with him practically not coming in on Fridays? How long can
he run around ragged like this? Yes these are the things that run
loops through my head on a daily basis. I am not worried about
me. I am worried about Eric and Ian.

Two Wolves – August 27, 2011

In church a few weeks ago our opening prayer was started off with a story, like it is every week. This story was about an old Indian man telling his grandson of the legend of every person having two wolves in him/her fighting to survive. One wolf represents all the good in us: our spirit God gave us all, joy, hope, love, dreams, gratitude, charity of our hearts, etc. The other wolf represents the opposite: greed, hate, fear, jealousy, etc. The grandson asked the grandfather, which one wins? The grandfather simply said, "The one you feed."

I feel like the "bad" wolf has been winning in me lately in so many ways and it has not been a good feeling at all. So many ugly feelings have been slowly creeping into me and I guess I kept feeding them until I felt like that was all I had in me.

Guilt: I have guilt over so many things. Things I didn't even know I could have guilt over. I have guilt over Ian. I feel guilty I can't be the mom I want to be to him. Some days I don't feel like playing, I don't feel like doing anything and I feel guilty about that. I have guilt about Eric. I feel guilty about me not being a healthy wife to help him more. I have guilt about myself. I feel guilty towards myself for not nurturing myself the way I think I should be, like painting more, cooking better, even just walking 30 minutes a day and so much more.

I have also felt jealousy towards almost everybody. I am jealous of their health, of their problems. I find myself wishing their problems were my only problems, jealous of their *easy* lives. The good wolf has tried to tell me that I don't know what their lives really are like, that I am doing all I can at this point, but hearing those little whispers of truth while hearing the giant roars of the negative. It is hard to hear them much less believe them. What makes it easier at times to hear one wolf over the other and only believe what that wolf is telling us?

I feel like some days I have the Will and Grace to do what needs to be done, to believe everything will be ok, to lean on God. Other days, well I don't. I don't know what happens during the night or when I wake up to make those days harder, to make me not believe it will all be ok, to make me not feel up to anything, to let me question God and His love for me. I don't know. I sure wish I did. Please pray that the good wolf continues to win in me, that I continue to have Grace and strength as the days get a little harder and harder. That I always know that God loves me, which I know he does but sometimes I just need a little reminding.

Chemo Chronicles 3.4 – 3.6 – August 29, 2011

I am not really sure if I should *count* Mondays in my chemo chronicles...being as it is a parp and not really chemo. But my thoughts are if I am getting poked in the port, it is a treatment. I am very happy to say that last Friday was SO much better than the first and today being my second Monday there; it is getting better every day. The nurses are just as kind and loving as the other office and I am starting to get know to them, which does make it easier. It seems my new schedule of events are: Friday – treatment. I am tired after treatment and am ready for bed around 7:30pm or 8:00pm. Saturday – sleep in and feel pretty good. I start going downhill around 4:00pm. Sunday – feel a little queasier. If I take medicine to make me not feel queasy I pass out for two and half to three hours. Monday – parp treatment and tired at night. I am tired but not down and out and each day seems to get a little better than the last. I have learned that going to bed around 8:00pm or 8:30pm is just the easiest way for me to feel better quicker. Not exciting but worth it.

We are heading out of town, so don't be alarmed when I don't write for over a week, the wolves haven't taken over! Speaking of the wolves, your comments mean a lot to me. I have taken these little pieces to heart and really know they are words of truth and love. I am trying to learn to be gentle with myself. I am hoping on vacation I can spend some time healing both physically and emotionally. And I need to remind myself we are all in a process of understanding and loving ourselves and each other. It doesn't just happen without work and more than likely even after doing a lot of work, it still takes more work.

Chemo Chronicle 3.7 and Trip – September 12, 2011

Friday was a long day, but a good day. I changed my appointment from 9:30am to 10:30am, so I could be the one to take Ian to his first day of school, which was a breeze. He didn't mind at all and although he wouldn't say it, I think he was a little excited to get back into a routine. Yes, he is my child. And this was my first Friday to fly solo. Eric needed to work while I was there so he could pick Ian up at 2:30pm. I saw Lisa, the PA. We just visited for a while which is so nice. My blood counts are holding pretty steady, my hemoglobin is creeping down. She said a small tidbit about if it gets down in the 8's we will talk about a blood transfusion, but it was 10.4 right now. Next Friday I will see Dr. H and also find out when my next CT scan will be. I am really hoping it is after next Fridays round. I read most of the day while I was there getting chemo. Eric made it up to visit me for a bit, and I was finally released to leave at 4:40pm.

It was a long day, but I held tight to God's plan anytime I would start getting anxious. I was trying hard to lean on God more during my difficult time instead of letting the craziness of all this get to me and beat me down. And I figured out yesterday that I would rather be there by myself and have Eric available to Ian versus him sitting up there with me. Both of us doing nothing and at least if he was at work during that time I didn't feel so guilty about all this because he could be with Ian after school.

Our trip to MI was nice, a little tiring but nice. We got home late Wednesday night and spent Thursday trying to get back in the swing of things around here. Ian had a fabulous time with his cousins. It was so cute to see them all together. He didn't really want Hanna hugging him which is hard to explain to a 2-year old that he just isn't a hugger and doesn't like people in "his" space. All turned out well though. I managed to get in a little relaxing and I followed my heart that was telling me to talk to Eric's older sister about some stuff that has been heavy on my heart lately. She is one of the strongest people I know in her faith and I just had some questions for her about well, my faith. I asked her how to stay strong in my faith and trust in God's plan when some days it all seems to be crumbling around me. It refilled my soul to hear her say that bad things happen to good people and that this isn't my fault. Eric tells me this all the time but to hear it from someone else is refreshing in a way I couldn't have imagined. It was great to see everyone, but it was nice to return home too.

Wonders & Worries – September 13, 2011

Well, I did it. I admitted to myself that maybe Ian needs Wonders and Worries. Today was the first visit. I had scheduled the first visit for a few weeks ago, then we decided to go to MI and I canceled. I almost canceled again because it is hard to admit that your child might need help. It is hard to admit that it is your situation that is causing your child to need help. It is hard to admit that this isn't ending any time soon and if he needs an outlet now, he will surely need one more in the months to come. So, I stuck with the appointment and we went today. Like anything new, I prepped Ian with as many details as he asked for and we went from there. He was a little confused because I called it a play date, so he thought he was going to Lexi's (our counselor's) house. I tried to explain that we were going to her work but "play date" stuck in his head and he was going with that.

She was great with him from the moment we got there. She complimented him on his crocs, which is one sure fire way to his heart. She gave him a snack out of the snack basket (score two for Lexi), and played a game with Skittles (she had his heart). AND she told me he looked just like me, so she had my heart too since I usually only hear that he looks like Eric! They went and played in the play room and I sat out in the waiting room and read a book. He later told me they played a game of "what makes you...." sad, happy, angry, etc. He made a family totem pole and played. She told me he did great. I am going to call her tomorrow to get more information from her. I don't want to talk about it with Ian right there. He listens to everything and would know I was talking about him. I was just really happy the first visit is over, he liked her and it seems like an easy thing to do. As far as doing something like this goes.

Cautiously Optimistic – September 26, 2011

Those are the exact words my nurse said Dr. H told her about my recent CT/Bone scans. The CT results are REALLY great. But I am also like Dr. H though, I am cautiously optimistic of the results since the experience last time. A great CT, two more rounds of chemo, a PET scan that was not what any of us thought, and growth of the tumors.

I am scared to get my hopes up too much, but I also want to be grateful for the blessing. It is an odd place. I prayed that the PET results (which I won't get for another seven weeks, after four more chemo treatments) mirror the CT results.

Tomorrow... - September 29, 2011

Tomorrow holds a lot of unknowns for me. What will Dr. H say about the latest CT scans? What exactly are we looking at here? Can I go ahead and schedule my PET scan in five or six weeks? (I REALLY hope so.) Can I go see a dentist? (I think one of my old cavity filling is coming out.) I have so many more questions. As much as I am looking forward to tomorrow to talk with Dr. H, I am NOT looking forward to chemo.

This break was so needed. Marci came to visit which was such a needed blessing. She knew I needed something and as soon as I said yes, she had her airplane ticket booked. She is a true blessing in my life. I needed my heart to get back into this fight. On days I feel like crap, my mind starts in with too many questions. How long can you really keep this up? How long can you feel like crap? How long can you let Eric do so much? What would happen if you didn't go to chemo again? But with this break, my heart could fight back to those questions and I knew this was God talking to my heart.

I am still struggling with what to eat. Meat kind of grosses me out lately, but if I am not eating meat I eat carbs and well, carbs aren't good for me because when I eat too many of them, my left foot swells up, aka inflamed which is not good. SO I really feel like I am in between a rock and a hard place with eating. Some days I really wish I could just not eat. My hair is starting to grow again too. It is weird to know that I am still on chemo and have this 5 o'clock shadow again. It is soft like baby hair too. I will report back with news after tomorrow's appointment. Please pray it is what I am hoping it is

A modern-day miracle – October 1, 2011
I know a lot of people don't believe the same as I believe-that God has a hand in everything. I do believe this and that is why I struggle so much with what has been going on. Lately though, I have started to believe more even though my circumstances are still the same. I still have cancer and chemo still sucks.

A lot has happened leading up to this moment. But the gist of it is that I found this book that was sent to me with the first go around of cancer. "Grace for Each Hour" by Mary Nelson. And honestly, I am not sure who even sent it and no one really seems to know if they sent it to me or not when I ask. I am not sure when, maybe two months ago, I had a very strong urge to start reading this book. It has spoken to me in ways I didn't know I wanted/needed to be spoken to.

"For I know the plans I have for you," says the Lord. "They are plans for good and not for disaster, to give you a future and a hope. In those days when you pray, I will listen. If you look for me in earnest, you will find me when you seek me. I will be found by you," says the Lord. "I will end your captivity and restore your fortunes. I will gather you out of the nations where I sent you and bring you home again to your own land." – Jeremiah 29:11-14

This was one of the many passages that began to take root in my heart, bring me peace and hope again; acceptance that no matter how much I didn't understand or want this situation. I have faith in the outcome, whatever it was to be. This book has changed the way I have been praying.

I have started praying for help. Flat out help with whatever it was that I need help with. I pray for help in surrendering all my worries over to Him. For help in listening to Him, for help in faith, for help in acceptance. I am done praying for me to be cured. I am done praying for me to understand the why in all this. I am done asking if He is mad at me. I am done praying about my cancer. I have started praying with a true abandonment of me. I am praying to be closer to Him, not because I am sick but because that is what I want. Marci told me a few weeks ago I seem to be at peace. That is when it hit me, I am at peace. I guess I really have handed it all over to God without me really knowing that I did.

Ok, but back to my modern day miracle, I do believe my heart changing in the way it has is a huge part of it happening when it did...now.

My CT scan from last week showed "no evidence of metastatic disease." This means that for all clinical purposes my cancer is in remission.

Now that is a true miracle.

I have been longing to see those words since this whole ordeal started again in March. I will long to see those words forever from every scan I ever get. I also found out yesterday that the trial I am in is now closed to new people. More proof to me that God had His hand in this the whole time. If the first chemo drug hadn't stopped working how and when it did, who knows if I would have been able to get into this trial...the trial drug that Eric has said all along he felt was the drug I needed to be on. Back to chemo, I still have to stay on chemo for a while. I have a PET scan at the first of November which will show a bigger picture and the stuff in my bones. If that comes back as clean as the CT, well I am still not sure what we will do. For right now, the only way to get the parp is to be on chemo because it isn't FDA approved. And, we all want me to keep getting the parp so for the time being I will still be on my Friday/Monday schedule for two weeks on and two weeks off. Thank you all for your support through all this. It does mean so much to me.

Please pray that I always see those words, "NO EVIDENCE OF DISEASE" from now on, on all my scans. Please pray the parp is approved soon. Please say thank you to God for this miracle.

A walking zombie… - October 8, 2011

I feel like a walking zombie, or what I assume a walking zombie feels like? It seems no matter how much I rest I am still exhausted. Not tired enough to sleep but too tired to actually do anything else. I have been on the verge of breaking down most of the week. These are the days when I question how much longer I can stay on chemo and feel like shit?

Yesterday was a long day. I got to office at 8:30am and left at 3:00pm. It was a zometa day.

My blood work showed that my neutrophils are super low, almost none existence. They were .3 and 1.5 is actually the lowest they like them to go. So pretty much right now I have no immune system which makes total sense that I feel like shit. Lisa, the PA and Lauren, the research nurse, came over to the chemo room talk to me about my counts being so low. They lowered my actual chemo yesterday in hopes of helping my body bounce back. Lisa also told me any sign of fever to call them immediately and to just lay low this weekend.

Lauren and I talked too. I asked her if she knew about other patients on the trial and if they were able to just do the parp and no chemo if they came back NED. She said yes she did and the trial takes it all on a case by case basis. I believe God sent her to talk to me yesterday and tell me that because I was starting to feel hopeless with the thought of this current chemo going on forever. I know nothing is set in stone and it all depends on my PET scan, which is scheduled for November 9th!

I feel a little broken down from this week. I am really praying that the Nuelasta shot on Monday helps me bounce back....even if it is just a little. It is weird to feel this broken down with the great news from last week, but I guess my counts don't care what the great news was.

Another hard one – October 16, 2011

This past week was a tough week for me, very tough. My fatigue seemed to take on a new life of its own and my mind wouldn't turn off. When I am trying to rest, I am not able to. I realized something this week though, I think depression has set in more. Which is such a weird thing because all I want to do is think of my last CT scan and the wonderful words on it, but I still have these hopeless feelings, lack of desire, and a sadness. I know it would seem that I could easily chalk these emotions/feelings up to chemo, but I have been depressed before and this feels all too familiar. I am going to find a talk therapist and talk to my oncologist to up my Lexapro. Going through this makes me wonder though, how many times does a person going through chemo or any major illness become depressed and it gets it chalked up to chemo side effects? Feeling depressed sucks. I tried to tell myself I could snap out of it or to stop feeling sorry for myself, but I know this is something I can't just snap out of on my own, just like I can't make my cancer go away without chemo.

Too Many – October 28, 2011

I need to stop reading so many murder mystery books because
all I can think to compare myself to right now is someone who
was buried alive and is crawling out of the grave. These past two
weeks have run me through a gamut of emotions, but I do feel
like I am out of the hole I have been buried in with maybe just a
foot left in there. Mentally, I am feeling better, especially taking
my Lexapro at the same time EVERY day. Yes, I must admit I wasn't
taking it daily. Dumb I know. Again, it was one of those things I
thought I could power through. I also made a therapy appointment
for November 8th, so I am hoping that will add to my arsenal of
defenses against this so called depression. I was told today that I
have to get a blood transfusion tomorrow because my red counts
are so low. Not really how I want to spend 6 hours of my Saturday,
but from what Eric and Gina have told me from what they have
read, it should really help with my energy levels. Here's praying for
that. These last few weeks have been a roller coaster of emotions,
but I do finally feel like I am back to a place of hope and desire to
continue on with this crap. I have had some wonderful days with
Ian, and those are the days I try to hold tight to when I am feeling
down. Unfortunately those aren't the thoughts that come through
when I am feeling down. The mind is a tricky thing and likes to play
mean tricks. Please continue to pray for us. Pray that the blood
transfusion is easy and does give me the energy boost I so need,
for Eric, and for Ian to continue to be a healthy and happy 4 year
old.

New blood and Halloween – November 2, 2011

The blood transfusion was LONG. We got there at 9:30am and left
at 4:00pm. Luckily I was in a private room, so we (Eric's mom and
I) hung out and watched TV. They gave me some Benadryl and I

passed out for about 2 hours. It was easy, but long. The million dollar question has been, "so, do you have more energy?" I would say yes a little.

Is it as much as I hoped it would be? No but I will take what I can get these days. We went to dinner Saturday night, I made it to Costco after church on Sunday with Eric and Ian, we went trick or treating on Monday night (even after chemo on Monday) so yes I guess I do have a little more energy. Am I ready to clean the house from top to bottom? No, but when am I ever?!?!

Halloween was a great time. Ian was Spiderman and only lasted maybe 3 minutes with his mask on, which I was fine with because he could hardly see with it on. We went trick or treating with all of our friends in the "hood" after a fun Halloween party. The kids had a blast and it was a lot of fun to see them all together. Ian did get a birdhouse for one of his treats; we are convinced the lady was cleaning out her garage. The other kids got other random treats from her house as well...very odd. I was very much looking forward to this being an off week. I needed an off week!

The Power of Prayer – November 8, 2011

I can see how others who continued to work through treatment said it was easier to have something to focus on. I have been praying for a way to help others in a way that didn't take too much energy or actually make me leave the house because I don't have much free time in between appointments and what free time I do have, I want to spend with Eric and Ian. The idea came to me last week to start a prayer request group for the Pink Ribbon Cowgirls. That is one thing I feel is lacking with this group – spiritual support. I do understand why they don't; there have to be different levels of support and their gig is getting people together to share stories, ideas, etc. But with that being said they don't say we, the group members, can't branch out and do things like this. I used to think

that God didn't want to hear our small prayers only the large ones.
But over time and study, I have learned that is not the case. He
wants to hear it all even the things that seem so small to us. And
I have personally learned, the more specific the prayers are the
easier it is for people to pray for you. I want all the girls in the PRC
to have as many prayers for them as I have had and continue to
have. Some of them don't have the wonderful support system I am
blessed with. I am excited to have this to organize. It is nice to have
something to do for others again. I am going to see how this goes,
get a feel for how many people get involved and the requests each
week and then open it up to others. How cool would it be to have
a FB page of just prayer requests? Then at any time, people could
go on there, pick a few requests and pray for them. I think it would
be awesome, but right now I know I can only manage this and am
thankful for this.

*"Therefore I tell you, whatever you ask for in prayer, believe that you
have received it, and it will be yours." – Mark 11:24*

First time for everything – November 11, 2011

Today was the first time I can say I wasn't happy with my doctor.
First the wonderfully great news, my PET/CT scan from Wednesday
shows no evidence of metastatic disease!! What we have all
been praying for all along. This is such a huge place to be and I
am truly thankful for this miracle. On the other hand, I am pissed
about today. It is a hard place to be to want to be so thankful for a
miracle yet pissed at my doctor. Long story short, she didn't seem
at all happy about the NED report from the PET scan, first thing
that I am pissed about. Then she kept saying *when* it comes back.
When NOT *If* but *When* which really pisses me off because she
doesn't know for sure it is going to come back. No one does. The
data might show others in my position, stage IV triple negative,

that it comes back after being in remission for some time, BUT it isn't 100%. That is what also pissed me off. She wants me to do another two full cycles of chemo so four more times of Friday/Monday treatments. Whatever, I am fine with that.

Then she said she hoped for me to be able to take a break for at least 6 months and *when* it came back, we would do more biopsies and possibly another treatment tactic. I zoned out at that point because honestly, I didn't want to listen to it anymore. I plan on proving her *when* thought completely wrong. Now as far as the parp being my maintenance, still nobody knows if that is possible. Another thing that pissed me off, I would think the drug company of the parp would have a plan for people getting to NED and them staying on only the parp and not chemo to show what wonderful things the parp does. I guess not. I am SO trying to get past all this, be in the moment of thankfulness of remission, get through these next four treatments and move on to something else. Ugh...cancer sucks. Please pray for my counts to stay up during these next four treatments and for a maintenance plan to be in place at the end of these four treatments, ideally the parp.

More News – November 15, 2011

One more answered prayer! I got a call from the trial nurse yesterday telling me that I can stay on the trial drug, the parp, without having to stay on chemo with it!! This is what I have been praying to hear. This is a chemo free maintenance! I will still have to go get "hooked up" Monday and Friday 2 weeks on, 1 week off, but it isn't full out chemo! I have to finish this current cycle of chemo on Friday, but after that, I will start just the parp. Eric has felt this is the path for me for some time now, and I know he wants the best for me. So I am going with all his research on the subject and saying this is the path for me.

Chemo chronicle 3.final – November 22, 2011

I was hoping with this being my final all out chemo, I could somehow slide through the side effects and just get on to life not on chemo.

I was wrong, really, really wrong. I have pretty much been in bed for 2 days. With no appetite and feeling nauseous every time I got up, the easiest way to deal with it was to sleep. And sleep I did. I feel better today and am praying I continue to feel better day by day. I guess this last chemo really wanted to show me what it could do. I get it ok, you are tough and no easy thing to contend with I wanted to yell at it. I am still in a little bit of shock and disbelief that was my last chemo. Now I feel like this is the time my faith has to carry me through just being on the BSI and not chemo. I know God put me in this position and I have to trust that even though it is scary. Yes, I am scared, very scared. Please pray for me to continue to be NED from here on out.

Maintenance – December 3, 2011

Well, yesterday was the first day of maintenance for me. So many emotions ran through me yesterday: excitement of not being on chemo, scared of not being on chemo, hesitant of what is to come and so much more.

It wasn't as easy of a day as I had hoped for though. After the blood work came back, I was told I need another blood transfusion. My red counts are lower than they have ever been, so I am writing this from a hospital bed waiting on my blood to arrive for the transfusion.

After getting my blood drawn at the hospital yesterday, I left after being there too long only to receive a phone call from the nurse who drew my blood telling me that she spelled my name wrong on the type and cross. And I needed to come back to the hospital to get more blood drawn. To say the least, I was pretty much done with yesterday. But my counts being SO low did explain why I had been so exhausted this past week in the evenings, exhausted as in going to bed to around 7:00pm and sleeping all night.

After seeing Dr. H again yesterday, all the frustrations I had from the last appointment was totally gone. She was so excited about me being on just the parp and told me I was her only patient on just the parp, and we were blazing new territory together. It was exciting, scary and so much more. She said she didn't know what the trial company was going to say about me being on just the parp, which explained so much from last time. Bring on life without chemo!

Just Parp – part 2 – December 11, 2011

Well, I can honestly say I am starting to feel better. A lot better. Yesterday I was still pretty tired, but I think that was from the zometa (bone stuff, yes, I still have to get that every 4 weeks). Today, I hung with the boys all day! It was great to be able to hang out with Eric and Ian, get stuff done around the house, play, go to dinner with friends and not feel like I was going to fall asleep midsentence. I have my parp tomorrow, bright and early so I can make it to Ian's Christmas program at 12:30pm. Then I am off until December 30th! What a wonderful Christmas present that will be and even better one to feel a little bit better every day. It is amazing how much I can tell a difference as each day passes as I get more energy back. It is amazing how much I can now tell the chemo was beating me up and how I don't ever want to go back there again. I pray every day a thankful prayer of the miracle He gave me and continues to give me daily.

It hits home… - December 20, 2011

Too many things have happened these past few days that makes my stomach turn and scares the crap out of me. One of our Pink Ribbon Cowgirls passed away. She was young, my age young, and had a 4 year-old son. My heart hurts for family and friends and especially her son. Then I just got an email update from another cowgirl. She stopped chemo September 15th and was free and clear of the C word. It is now back and she has to start chemo again.

I don't get it.

I just don't get it.

I do so good at thinking I am doing good and thinking I have it all under control and then something like this happens and all I can think is how this could so easily be me.

It is a fine line I am trying not to cross, thinking about these people, their situations, their hurt and in turn thinking "what if" that is me again?

It could so easily be me again. It sucks, CANCER SUCKS!!!

2012

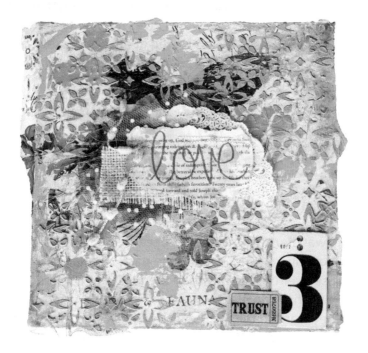

Same song and dance… - January 15, 2012

I haven't had much excitement going on lately which I am NOT complaining about! Just not anything notable to blog about, so I apologize for the lack of writing.

Things are going really well. I am feeling a little better every day, my hair is growing (almost long enough to not look like "cancer hair"), we bought an elliptical and I am doing that at least 30 minutes a day (it is a start…nowhere near what I was doing before chemo, but I am trying to learn to give myself a break… trying), doing a weekly bible study with some of my friends which I completely love studying with them, started painting/crafting again which is bringing me so much peace and happiness. It is with all these wonderful things going on that my upcoming PET scan scares the heck out of me.

Dr. H told me a few weeks ago she doesn't expect anything to change on it from the last one which gives me great comfort, but I would be lying if I said I wasn't scared at all. Of course I am. I am trying to give that fear over to God, to let myself remember He is in ultimate control but it is hard not to worry.

My scan is this coming Wednesday. Please pray that it is shows no evidence of disease.

Scan News…- January 20, 2012

Honestly, I was starting to freak out because I hadn't heard anything from anyone in 2 days. In the past, I had usually heard my scan results either the day of or the next day. My mind starts playing mean tricks on me. I start to think that they aren't calling because they want to tell me the news while I was there and that had to mean bad news. WRONG. Scans shows nothing, nada, zilch! I am still NED!!!!It turns out Dr. H's nurse is out of town this week and she is the one who always emails and calls me, we are tight like that! But with her being out of town, things fell through the cracks, as Lisa told me, and she felt horrible that I hadn't gotten my results. No one needed to feel bad, I just needed to hear that my report was boring. I like boring.

A bit of catch up – February 10, 2012

 Wow, time really does fly when you are having fun, I guess…or I just haven't felt like writing – maybe a little of both!

The three of us, Eric, Ian and myself, went on a cruise to Mexico and had a great time being our little family of 3.

Treatment started up again today. I saw Dr. H, and asked her a few questions that I had been wondering about lately. I wanted to get more details on my latest PET scan and the details were that there aren't ANY details to get! I asked her if my bones were still lighting up in the scan and NOPE they weren't, for those of you who aren't versed in PET *talk* no light up means no uptake which means no cancer! She told me I am NED NED, double NED! I really almost fell out of my chair when she told me this. I didn't expect to hear this absolutely great news. I also asked her if I would stay on this parp indefinitely, and the answer is yes, well kind of. This parp is still not FDA approved, so I am still in a trial. As long as the trial people still feel like I am helping their cause, I will still get the medicine. But like she said, I couldn't be helping them anymore than I was. She wasn't concerned that I would be kicked out and not get the parp.

I am still in awe of the miracle that has taken place within me both physically and spiritually this past year. I think about all the tiny little details that God had to line up to make this happen...and it not only happened, it happened in a HUGE way! I will get a CT in mid-March, still get my treatment every Monday and Friday and continue to carry on with life and be thankful for all the tiny little details that God doesn't ever overlook.

Blank slate... - February 16, 2012

Too many days I feel like my head is a blank slate. I can be in the middle of a conversation and literally have no idea what I was just talking about, I forget simple words, if I don't write an appointment down there is no way I will remember it. I used to be able to remember the most random appointments, certain memories are just gone. Eric will ask me if I remember something and I don't, or I only remember little pieces of it. It is so bizarre what I do and don't remember, how chemo brain affects me a

little bit different daily. I feel socially awkward when I am just
left blank...with no idea of what was being said one second ago.
Fortunately my family and friends are awesome and let me ask
them the same question multiple times, sometimes daily (or more)
for a week or so until I realize we have talked about it, but then I
still don't remember the answer.

Now I preface a lot of questions with, "I might have already asked
you this." Now that I don't look like "cancer" anymore aka, my
hair is growing out past the point of, *yep, she was bald at some
point*, and my skin isn't grey and ashy. Strangers do look at me like
I might be a little bit crazy, mostly when I am ordering something
or asking for help in a store because 9 times out of 10, I get to the
person I need to speak with and have no idea what it is I want to
order or ask about. Maybe they think I am drunk, who knows? And
maybe they don't really notice anything and it is just me thinking it
is a much bigger deal than it actually is, kind of doubt it but could
be?!?!

A little bit of this...a dash of that – February 24, 2012

A little bit of this...a dash of that is what makes up my life, and I
feel truly blessed every day for all those this and thats. Things are...
dare I say...normal? Around here lately....well, getting there. My
hair is growing back which I love. I never minded being bald, but I
do enjoy having hair versus no hair! It is growing back light brown,
straight, and soft with a cowlick in front. Last time it came back
(yes, it is weird to me to think this is the second time in my adult
life I have a whole new head of hair) it was black and curly. I have
always had dark brown hair, so it being this light is taking some
getting used to.

I am really able to work out again. We got an elliptical at the house and I have been doing that at least 30 minutes daily, some days I do 45-50 minutes. I forgot how good it feels to sweat and to be sore and just feel active. I did Zumba this week and loved it. Now, don't get me wrong, chemo didn't give me some unexplained rhythm I wasn't born with, I still look like a white girl with no moves, but it was a much better workout than I thought and I had a great time listening to the music and letting go. I still need to go to bed early, not as early as I was but I am usually asleep by 9:00pm (unless I drink coffee at 5:00 in the evening, no, not a good idea...even Ambien won't put me to sleep after that!) I thank God daily, multiple times a day, for all the blessings in my life. I might be on maintenance forever (which honestly, I pray that I am...that way I know I am cancer free), have to go in two times a week for infusion, but honestly, it doesn't matter. I am cancer free and have a truly blessed life from every which way.

I believe – February 29, 2012

I believe God has a plan and a purpose for each and every one of us. I believe it is up to each one of us to listen to His *instructions*, *tips*, *hints*, or whatever you want to call them and to do something with them. I believe He gives us all talents and projects to carry out in our lifetime in order to help each other, spread love, kindness, grace, hope and so much more. I believe it is our duty, as children of God, to try to love each other as He loves us. I believe the events in our lives are all planned out by Him to reach a certain outcome. I believe He speaks directly to our hearts all the time. I believe it is our duty to love and praise Him, to tell others the peace, love, comfort He gives us. I believe He has been putting little tidbits of information, of other people's inspirations, other people in my life all along to help me know that what I have started painting can help people, help them love Him more, help them heal, help them embrace life, love and God. I have found comfort and healing in painting. I have had several people ask me to do commission work, which at first I was scared and didn't know, but decided to take a leap of faith and do it! I am going to do this, I am going to paint pictures of love and hopefully sell them too!

Cheers...where everybody knows your name – March 4, 2012

I don't necessarily want to go, but I do feel like with all my treatment appointments, visiting my doctor, her nurses, the receptionist, the schedulers, I know everyone there and surprisingly enough, they all know my name too. I guess not too surprising...I am there twice a week. Eric went with me Friday for a bit. He was feeling guilty for not being able to come more often, but I tell him all the time that I am good to go, they all take great care of me and it is like Cheers in there, we all know each other's stories and they will always give you the good stuff!

One year ago... - March 8, 2012

I got the call that I will never forget. "Renee, Dr H. wants to see you today, there is something showing up on your CT scan." My world...our world promptly started spinning out of control. I had no idea what was in store for me, I had no idea what the next weeks would hold, much less the next whole year...but, here we are, one year later and now I know. I know I can do this. I can and will fight for my life with every ounce of my being. I know how truly blessed I am. My friends and family totally rallied around us, put up a protective barrier and took care of us...they took care of me when I was sure I couldn't do chemo anymore, when I was sure my Lexapro was not working just right, when I had nothing left to give them, they took care of me. I know what an amazing husband I have...I knew this before, but now I KNOW it! He has been my rock in so many ways. He never once asked more of me than what I was able to give, heck, he never even asked anything from me. I know that Ian's smiles, hugs and kisses...his presence can cure a lot of pain and heartache without him even realizing what he is doing.

I know that miracles do happen...I am one. I know that God has me covered in love and is with me every single step of the way, with or without cancer. I know now what true inner peace feels like and I know God gives me that inner peace. I know now what truly turning something over to God is like and how to 100% depend on Him. I know now that I am extremely grateful for being able to fold clothes, unload the dishwasher, do routine chores....it is a HUGE blessing to feel like doing that stuff....both physically and mentally. I know now to tell everyone in my life what they mean to me, how much I love them, all the time...if I want to hear it from them then they want to hear it from me. I know I do like having hair versus not – I LOVE IT! I know that I don't want to know what it is like to have it grow in a third time. I know painting fills my soul with goodness. I know that I can honestly say, stage IV, stage IV...I've got this. I can't wait to see what the next year has in store for us and what another year full of blessing will teach me.

Crystal clear... - March 18, 2012

Thank you God for another crystal clear CT scan this time around and always. I had a CT scan on Thursday and whoop whoop – I am still NED!! I try so hard not to stress over these scans, but little thoughts always seem to seep into my mind. I pray hard for God to change my heart to trust He is handling this. But my silly mind wants to take over.

We had an AWESOME spring break this past week. Eric's parents have been in town, so Ian has been in real vacation mode! We went to Sea World on Wednesday and had a fabulous time. It was overcast and a little misty in the morning, so I think that kept the big crowds away. Ian was tall enough to ride some rides and he loved it! Eric and I even rode the Steel Eel and The Great White. I haven't ridden a rollercoaster since Ian was born. I loved the Steel Eel, the Great White kind of sent me over the edge with all the loops and turns. I needed some dip-n-dots to settle my stomach! I did well on my eating while there. Had a salad for lunch and splurged on the dip-n-dots, which Ian and Eric ate at least half of, so I didn't feel that bad!

Thwack... - March 23, 2012

I *hit a wall* last night. It has been a long time since I needed to go lay down at 6:30pm and stay in bed for the night. Granted Eric and I watched some TV and I didn't go to sleep until 10:00pm, but I was exhausted last night. It is times like that that I am reminded I am still in treatment, my body still gets worn down easily and I need to listen to it and know when to say enough, I am done. So that is what I did last night. I SO wanted to get a canvas done to deliver today, but I just couldn't. Oh well, there is today! I think it had to do with my nerves. Just when I get used to not going to treatments, my start of the next two week cycle rolls around and the Thursday night before, I am always a nervous wreck. I have no idea why. I have to remember to be gentle with my body. It is going through a lot and it does take good care of me. We are going to Fort Worth this weekend to hang out with the family. I am really looking forward to it! I think Ian can't see straight he is so excited about it! I love seeing him with his cousins. It brings pure joy to my heart!

Learning to love again...- April 2, 2011

One thing I have noticed with this whole cancer gig is that no one really ever talks about the things we want to talk about. Actually I have noticed that in life, we all pretend everything is great, life is great, there are no hardships, but there are hardships and sometimes things just suck and need to be talked about.

So here it goes, I haven't been physically able to have intercourse since last May. It hurt so bad I thought I was going to cry. Then I just gave up on trying. I want to be able to have relations with my husband. There had been a lot of talk on the Pink Ribbon Cowgirls site about lubrications and how we all (us cancer girls) thought this was our problem, no hormones meant no lubrication.

Then one of our fellow cowgirls told us she went to pelvic floor physical therapy. At first, I was like what in the hell are you talking about? She and I are friends, so I messaged her to ask her some questions. Then we went to lunch, and I quizzed her more about pelvic floor therapy. She told me it wasn't as crazy weird as it sounds. She said it was just like going to a gynecologist, and it was just another appointment.

So I decided what the heck, I needed help with my girl parts hurting during intercourse. I emailed my doctor to get a prescription for it. Who knows what she thought after my email. I rambled on that I needed to go to sex therapy and needed a prescription for it and one of my friends went, who isn't her patient but another doctor's patient and blah, blah, blah. She wrote back, here is a prescription for Pelvic Floor PT. *Sweet, I was in!* My first appointment was last week.

Sara, my PT, was awesome. She was very personable, explained everything to me and made me not feel like a complete weirdo for needing to be there. She explained that so many times people think painful sex is a lube problem and WAY too many times, people think there is nothing to be done about it. But she assured me there was something to be done. When I left last week, I joked and said, yeah, I am fixable!! She told me I was completely fixable. A good tip for you women out there, use Coconut Oil for lubrication...cheap, easy and healthy! So, my homework is to use dilators daily to expand me. She told me I might need to do this for two to three months...I guess it is true what they say, use it or lose it.

This week when I went she did a deep tissue massage on the fibers of the body that are all connected (no, I can't remember the name and google isn't helping me any). She massaged my lower abdomen and inner thighs and it freaking HURT. She told me it wouldn't feel good and it would leave bruising and yes indeed it did. This was to help "break up" the tissue and make it more expandable. From now on, she said she would do the deep tissue massage, and then when I was ready, I would start working on Kegels. I am super excited though because I was telling Dr. H's nurse last week about this (I am the first patient they have sent there) and she asked me today how it was going and that she wanted to start sending more people there. I think this totally needs to be an option for women and not just be told to use an estrogen cream and *relax*.

Truly... - May 4, 2012

"I know the plans I have for you, declares the Lord, plans to prosper you and not to harm you, plans to give you hope and a future." – *Jeremiah 29:11*

It always amazes me when I hear others talking about wanting to get on the drug I am on, the parp. It truly amazes me when I think about all the plans God had laid out for me WAY before I knew what was going to happen. Way before I was even born. It truly amazes me that my first chemo stopped working right when it did, that the parp trial was open, that I got in with NO effort, that the trial was/is available right here in Austin, that the parp people emailed Dr. H to tell her they want me to have an endless parp supply and the endless things that were laid out for me before I ever even thought about cancer. I had a PET scan yesterday and got my results today. "Absolutely boring" is what she told me. I told her I will take boring any day when we are reading scans. Six months as "NED" No Evidence Of Disease as a triple negative stage IV person is kind of unheard of. And you know what I say to that, well...*what does 10 years, then 20 years, then 50 years as a "NED Triple Negative Stage IV" look like?? Oh, it looks like ME!!*

34... - May 12, 2012

34...when I was "younger" I looked at 34 as old. I now look at 34 and think there is still so much more to come.

I just watched a movie called "We Bought a Zoo" and there was a line in it that I think we all need to live by, "you only need to be courageous for 20 seconds." If you blow it and make yourself look like a fool, well it is only 20 seconds. But it might be magical; all your dreams could come true from that 20 seconds of courage. 20 seconds of courage.

I feel with every birthday I get a little more courageous, a little more me. A little more ready to fully live. In my 34th year, I want to:

Stay cancer free

Love my family and friends as much as possible

Stay in the moment

Be brave and step out of my comfort zone with my art

Send my art to people

Go into shops to ask them to sell my art

Travel...a lot. We are going to Florida in May, Michigan in June, Schlitterbahn in July, California in August, the beach sometime in October and there is a Disney cruise talk going on with my mom! We are planning a Virgin Isle trip with Eric's family for next February, now that is what I am talking about! I REALLY want to get an RV and travel around and do craft shows. How cool would that be?

Swim a mile straight even if it is with a snorkel. I don't care, I can't get my stroke/breath down.

Read my bible daily even it is only for one minute, I want to be able to say, "I have read my bible EVERYDAY since I turned 34" (I totally stole this idea from Eric!)

Paint everyday

From my 34th year...I want to be able to look back on it when I am 90 years old and say, yes, that was the year I really learned to live... bravely.

Through me...Use Me – May 13, 2012

I try to live my daily life as an expression of God, be as kind, compassionate, giving, forgiving, and loving as Jesus. To truly listen to what He is asking me to do and most importantly, DO IT!

I have been praying for a new way to serve my church since I can no longer be an angel to the pre-k class (too many kids plus too many germs plus mama going through chemo equals not good!) So here it was a chance for me to help. The youth group needed money for a mission trip they were working for the summer. I asked them if they would be interested in me selling my canvases on their behalf and 50% of the proceeds would go to them. They were delighted to accept! And, I did it! I was nervous, but I kept asking God to calm me, and He kept assuring me he had the details covered and not to worry about it! It was great. It was beautiful day full of life and love! And, it was a huge success! I went in with three boxes full of canvases and left with a half a box! From a book: "Jesus, I don't want to fall short of the potential you put in me. Express yourself fully through me and in me."

All out of words – May 16, 2012

Ian: Mommy, how many long is 3 hours?

Me: 180 minutes.

Ian: How long is 5 hours?

Me: 300 minutes.

Ian: How long is infinity?

Me: Forever.

Ian: If you love Jesus, will you still die?

Me: Yes.

Ian: My friend said you won't die if you love Jesus?

Me: They are wrong.

Ian: Is God or infinity bigger?

Me: God is infinity.

Ian: What is infinity plus one?

Me: Infinity.

Ian: Is God everywhere?

Me: Yes.

Ian: Even standing on top of our heads?

Me: Sure, I guess that counts as everywhere.

Ian: When do we get to go up to Oma and grandpa's again?

Me: At the end of June...about 6 weeks.

Ian: How many days?

Me: Well a week has 7 days, so 6 times 7 is 42...42 days.

Ian: What is God doing right now?

Me: Loving us.

Ian: Oh!

Me: Baby, mommy is all out of words.

Ian: Well, you just said words, so you must not be all out.

He is four and a half years old. What are our conversations going to be like when he is 7? Full out math equations and philosophy discussions??

Art Bra – May 21, 2012

Art Bra is put on by the BCRC – Breast Cancer Resource Center here in Austin. I have been a part of this group from day 1 of my getting diagnosed and my best friend called them on my behalf to ask for help. Art Bra Austin, BCRC's Signature Fundraiser, is a runway show featuring an eclectic collection of art bras modeled by BCRC clients, reflecting the diversity of the women we serve. The array of Art Bras featured in the live and silent auctions are submitted by professional artists and designers, celebrities, organizations, and supporters of BCRC. On May 21, 2012, I was one of the models.

Oh what a magical night...magical. The energy in the room was intense, a great intense throughout everyone there. You could feel the love all around, from us modeling, to all the hard work volunteers put into it to make it so great, the family, friends, our doctors...the room was filled with love, pure and simple. But most of all the room was filled with lots of survivors showing off their confidence!

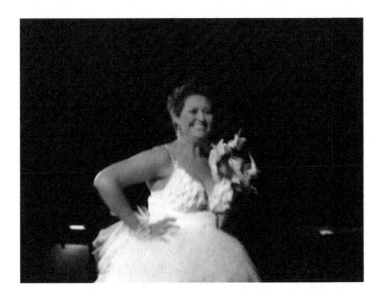

Celebrate – June 5, 2012

Our preacher preached about celebration on Sunday. How we
are really good at celebrating BIG things in our lives, holidays,
birthdays, milestones, promotions, etc. And those are all great
things to celebrate but what about all the small things that
make up our days, our weeks, our lives. All the small things that
make our hearts bust in excitement but we don't celebrate them
because we don't feel they are "big enough" for celebration? A
Psalm for Thanksgiving,

"Shout joyfully to the Lord, all the earth." – Psalms 100:1

It doesn't say only for big things. I have started then stopped,
started then stopped, started...keeping a gratitude journal. I want
to turn this into a celebration journal too. To write down my small
victories to celebrate daily and no that doesn't mean celebrate
with a glass of wine and a cupcake. I wish! Just celebrate! Say it
out loud that I am proud of something I did, recognize any and all
achievements. Celebrate with myself, with Eric, my friends, family,
strangers. I have gotten better celebrating my NED (NO evidence
of disease) status. When someone asks me how I am without
missing a beat I almost shout wonderfully great. Still NED, still
feeling great! I no longer have a *but, not sure,* or *eh* in there. There
is no room for that with NED! I need to get better at celebrating
my small victories with life, home life, business. I think I should
celebrate the nights I cook dinner; when all the laundry is done;
having canvas 6 orders waiting for me to do; when Ian helps me
clean up his stuff. It is these things that are life and should be
celebrated. What can you celebrate today, big or small??

Party Barge - June 10, 2012

June was a great month. We rented a double-decker party barge on Lake Travis to have a great big thank you party for all of our friends and kids who have helped us so much along this path. It was a blast! The kids were drunk on fun and tiredness. The adults were drunk on good time with friends.

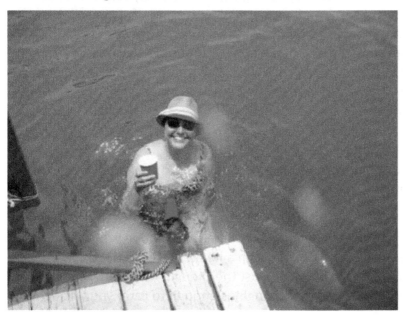

4 Steps – June 25, 2012

Today we had a guest speaker at church and he was great. He was talking about "interesting times." How these are the times that God uses to grow us. And we (as free-will individuals) have the choice to make every day (especially in "interesting times") if we are going to be in the moment joyfully or pissed off (no, he didn't use these words) because either way, we are going to stay in the moment until it passes.

"A joyful heart makes a cheerful face; but when the heart is sad, the spirit is broken." – Proverbs 15:13

I have had some anxiety lately. There have been a lot of "interesting times" happening with some of my cancer friends. Reoccurrences, hospital stays and worse and of course all these lead me to play the "what if" game. Then my head gets so wrapped up in that what if game, it is hard for my heart to get the truth back out to me. I AM NED (NO evidence of disease)...end of story...that is all I need to know for today that is all I have is today, today.

So our speaker spoke on 4 steps to get us out of our heads when it all comes crashing down and get us back to our heart to where we can hear God and listen.

Step 1. Hope on a foundation of gratitude "Hope is the dream of someone awake." Hope is such a beautiful thing. Hope can truly get you through SO much. Just the thought of it being a tiny bit better is hope and that thought is enough to carry you through.

Step 2. Faith. Trust and believe in something you don't see. I don't believe we don't see God. I believe we can choose to see Him in everything. But I know it takes faith to believe in His love for us, His hand reaching out to you in the dark.

Step 3. Joy. When your heart shows up on your face. Our speaker was given 6 months to live over a year ago. He said it all with his JOY to be up there, speaking, showing us. He said, "We all only know we have today so we need to dance."

Step 4. Love. Love is all around us all the time. It is up to us to look for it, feel it, and return it, BUT it is always around us.

All of these are on a foundation of gratitude. Gratitude for what we have. Not longing for what we want. Even in the midst of dark, dark times, we have SO much to be thankful for.

When I was smack in the middle of chemo and I honestly thought I couldn't do one more treatment, I prayed and saw this vision in my head. A BIG canyon, I was on one side and Eric and Ian were on the other. God told me NOT to look down, look only ahead to them. I did just as He said, and He held my hand all the way across the canyon to them. I realized then that I am alive, I always have Him there to hold my hand, I have an AWESOME family and friends, I have a talent that lets me speak my heart, Eric is able to provide for us in an amazing way, etc, etc, etc, etc. The list could seriously go on forever. That is when it hit me; I have to be thankful for what I have not long for what I want. I have to remember this every day. I know we each need to remember this every day. I know we all are going through our own times some more interesting than others, but there is something in your situation that you can be grateful for find it and hold on it.

Family Pictures – July 7, 2012

We had family pictures done by a friend in the neighborhood. Oh, they turned out so great.

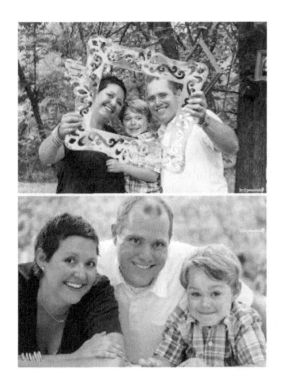

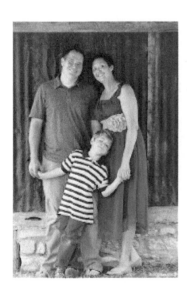

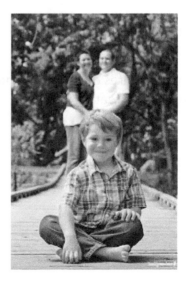

Our first fight… - July 20, 2012

I am not even sure you would call it a fight, but Ian and I had it out.

It was our first time that I am pretty sure we both broke each other's hearts.

It was time to clean out all the "stuff" we had been holding onto for way too long.

Ian's 5th birthday is coming up and I know he will be getting more stuff. So I started digging stuff out of the closet to sell on craigslist. We have been reading a book about a garage sale.

He seemed to get the idea.

We made piles: pile to put on craigslist, pile to keep, and pile to think about.

We went through the piles again and settled on what items were going where.

I started getting rid of the stuff in the to-go pile.

It was all great until he noticed something that was gone…a boat that he hadn't played with in months.

"Mommy, how could you do this to me? I didn't say I wanted to sell that. I earned that as a prize. (Which yes he did – FOR POTTY TRAINING – how did he even remember this?!?!?!?) You did this on purpose….."And on, and on, and on. It was bad. My heart was broken. I tried to explain to him that no, I didn't do this on purpose. That no, it was never my intention to hurt him. That no, even though he was mad at me, he was not allowed to speak to me in this way. That no, he did NOT get to keep the new toys if we got the boat back. That no, I couldn't take the crying anymore. He was hurt, mad and confused. I was hurt and mad. So what happened? I made him a deal. I bought a new boat from Amazon (although he thinks I just got it back from the guy who bought it) and I made him take his toys that he bought with the money from the boat sale back. I felt like a failure, like the lesson went unlearned because I caved, but I just couldn't fight anymore. And to add insult to injury, Ian told Gina, "Did you know that my mommy sold my very favorite toy? My favorite boat, she sold it." I told him he better play with this damn boat EVERYDAY!

I forget… July 29, 2012

I forget so easily how blessed we are to have me feel good 95% of the time.

I forget so easily how feeling like crap is a total drain on me mentally and physically.

I forget so easily how feeling like crap is a total drain on Eric and Ian.

I forget so easily how easy it is to fall into a hole.

I forget so easily how hard it is to pull myself out of that hole.

I forget so easily how hard it is to get out of bed when your body aches, when you are so tired for no good reason (well, beyond the chemo just received 24 hours earlier), when your desire for the day is gone.

I forget so easily how hard it really is to go through chemo.

I forget so easily because I am blessed beyond my own comprehension.

I am blessed to only have to feel like this once every 6 weeks instead of 4 days out of 7.

I never want to forget my blessings.

I never want to have to fully remember how bad full out chemo really is.

I never want to forget how utterly precious life is.

The inevitable… - August 16, 2012

It happened.

I didn't realize how hard it would be to deal with.

I didn't realize how quick it can happen.

I didn't realize the hole that would be left in my heart.

I guess when I started making friends with a bunch of cancer chicks, I should have known it was inevitable.

I should have known it would really suck.

I should have known it would rip my heart out into a million little pieces. I should have known all the questions would instantly start playing in my head, why her, why not me, what about her family, her husband, her two little boys, why does my treatment work and not hers?

The questions won't stop.

I met Kristi after I was diagnosed as Stage IV. I was at Costco with Ian and my in-laws when someone came up to me and asked me if I was Renee. I am sure the look on my face was a little taken aback, but then she quickly explained that she was a Pink Ribbon Cowgirl and well I didn't have any hair. I guess put two and two together and you get an odd meeting in Costco.

We instantly hit it off. She was funny, friendly and kind, my kind of girl. Then we got to know each other on a level not many people will ever know each other on, over many rounds of chemo. Yes it is true; we cancer chicks really get to know one another over chemo. We texted each other to see if we would be there at the same time, we wheel our bags of chemo around the infusion room to chat with each other, we get to hug each other when we get a great scan, we were there for each other when the scan wasn't what we hoped and prayed for. All of this in this surreal room filled with disease and more love than one would imagine. I was able to go see her in the hospital a few times. It was great to see her with her other friends, to see her as her, not as a cancer patient. I didn't get to say goodbye to her though. I was planning on going to see her tomorrow after my treatment as I was out of town until tonight...

It sucks. Cancer sucks. It is a real slap in the face. It is a real eye-opener, tomorrow is not a guarantee for anyone and it is heartbreaking.

To my sweet friend Kristi, I am sorry I didn't get to say goodbye. I am sorry you had cancer. I am sorry it took you away from us way too soon. I am sorry to your sweet husband and precious boys. I am sorry to your family and friends who loved you so much. You will be missed and you are oh so loved by so many.

The Aftermath... - August 18, 2012

While driving home from the funeral today, several things occurred to me:

We are a bunch of 30 and 40 year old people there to celebrate Kristi's life. But the thing is a bunch of 30 and 40 year olds shouldn't have to be at a funeral of another 40 year old. It was a heart breaking experience. Seeing her life in pictures, hearing the thoughts of her loved ones makes me realize so much. The small things that we spend SO much time and energy on...DO.NOT. MATTER. In the end, the stress we put on ourselves to have a perfect house, to have a perfect body, to have the perfect car. The standards we set for ourselves, none of it matters. When it is all said and done, the only thing that really matters is love, love for God, love for family, love for friends, love for each other. And to see Kristi in all those pictures with her family and friends made me realize that our lives are one big series of stories that we should strive to share with each other. Our lives are meant to be lived with family and friends. Our lives are meant to be shared with each other. I really want to look at the priorities I have had lately. I want Eric to look at his. I want to remember to live and deeply love every day. I want to remember the precious gift God gives us to live with our loved ones and to cherish the time here and to love as much as I can.

My sweet Ian – on your 5th birthday – August 24, 2012

Let me go ahead and get it out of the way. I can NOT believe you are 5, seriously, can NOT believe it. Where has the time gone? As sad as I am that you are growing up so fast, I am all that proud and more of what a truly wonderful person you are and are continuing to become. While over at a friend's house the other day you were calling me mom instead of mommy, then you whispered to me that you will call me mommy in secret. At least you are telling me your secrets! You have a wonderful outlook on life, one that is infectious. When I tell you that you can do something for 10 minutes, you say, "Well, at least it is more than 9!" And I always tell you that, "it is what it is" and one day you replied, "and it isn't what it isn't." You have a grasp on life much deeper than many adults I know. You live with a joy from deep down in your soul. You are so kind and caring to everyone. I tell you if someone hits you that you are allowed to hit them back and 9 times out of 10 you don't. You tell me you don't want to hurt them back. You teach so much everyday about kindness and love. You quiz me and daddy about God and Heaven all the time and are starting to understand that God is infinite and His love goes on forever. You asked me the other day if you were *my everything*, yes my sweetie, yes you are.

You continue to amaze me daily with your math in your head ability, you get that from me! The whole time we are driving, we are asking each other math questions. You have addition and subtraction pretty much down and we are starting to work on multiplication. You love math, love it. You are really starting to be interested in reading. You ask me specifically what everything says and are starting to sound out words. Your teachers from pre-k and gymnastics tell me what a wonderful friend you are to all, how well you listen and follow the rules and how kind and funny you are! You love performing magic tricks while daddy and I watch intently at all your shows! You haven't figured out how not to tell the secret of the trick though!

You still LOVE when daddy gets home! By 5:30pm, you and I are ready for a little break and you are ready to rumble with daddy! You LOVE to play board games, and we spend a majority of our time together doing just that. Right now you love, "guess who" "operation" "memory" (which you honestly win at) and "connect four." You are a gaming fool, but that is really ok with me! I don't cut you any slack with the rules. Sometimes you try to pull one over on me, but most of the time you do follow the rules and we are good to go! You still love Skylanders and have collected them all. You are currently saving up money to buy the new giants game that comes out in October! You are starting to like to play school, ninja school that is. You like to be the master who teaches me how to do certain ninja routines. It is so funny to watch! I really can't believe you are 5. It is amazing to see what a wonderful person you have become in these past 5 years. I can't wait to see who you are in the next 5 years.

I love you my sweetness,

Mommy

SO - September 1, 2012

I have tried to come up with witty titles and well, the only one I am able to think of is: Third time's the charm?!?!

Yesterday was a day like no other. Ian and I were running errands and after our stop at Pier One, we were walking down the stairs to go to Party City to start looking at Halloween stuff, because you know why wouldn't we start looking and thinking about Halloween costumes two months in advance?! Exactly!

While walking down the stairs my right side kind of went numb. Not all the way numb but for me to get it to work, I had to think the thought "move right foot" over and over to get it to move. After almost falling down the stairs, I called Eric right away because I was thinking driving wasn't the best idea! Eric and I thought it might be from low blood sugar, so we went to get some lunch. At lunch, the numbness got worse and my right foot was heavy. I could still move it, but it was heavy and weird. I called Dr. H and she said go to the ER now.

YIKES that freaked me out.

We got to the ER, Dr. H had already called, so we were able to go right back. Hey, I guess having an oncologist that rocks has its perks?!

Eric left me there and took Ian over to Teri's because we had no idea how long we would be there and let's just say a five year old in the ER doesn't equal happiness. They did an immediate EKG then Dr. H ordered an MRI. We waited for the MRI results.

The ER doctor came in to give us the news.

It was definitely NOT what we were expecting. ER doctor told me that there is a mass in my brain.

Not sure why, but every time I get this kind of news, I expect the doctor to pause and say, "Just Kidding...you are good to go...get on out of here."

I waited for it.

I prayed for it.

For him to say those next few lines...he didn't.

So me and Eric did what we do, we hugged, we cried, we said it sucks, we hugged some more then we shook it off, pulled on our brave pants and asked what comes next? Where do we go from here? The neurosurgeon came in to talk to us (I thought he was at the hospital and just stopped by, but come to find out from Dr. H this morning, she called him yesterday and asked him to stop by to talk to us) score 14,857 for Dr. H being awesome! He showed us the MRI and the mass is on the back of my brain. It was two to three cm large and mostly liquid. As far as having a mass on the brain goes, this one was in a REALLY good place. It wasn't in a place that could affect memory, speech, personality, body movement, etc. Gina told me they better not take the crazy out of me. I will still be me just without a piece of my brain.

Next steps: PET scan; consult with brain doctor and surgery on Thursday or Friday.

In the meantime, mom and Tammy are flying in today. Rachele and dad will be here for surgery. Eric's parents want to come also, but I think we will have them wait a few weeks to help with post-op.

Dr. H called to touch base with me this morning. She said if I was to have to get another tumor, this is the best place to get one. It could be cut out, radiated and good to go. She laughed and said it sounds weird, but more than anything this was just a major inconvenience. Which I tell her all the time saying cancer is just one big pain in my ass. If you are the praying type, will you please pray for a few things:

Dr. H gets approval for me to stay on BSI (the trial drug, they MIGHT see this as me being not NED, but she said that is stupid because systemically, I am NED. None of the chemo drugs I have had can cross the blood brain barrier...therefore; there has been no way for any drugs to get to my brain.)

Surgery is easy and I don't miss any of my brain

Body PET shows no evidence of disease

I know Eric and I have the strength and grace to make it through this bump in the road. We are faithful that God is good and He does have a bigger plan for us. Does that make it suck any less? No, it still sucks, but it will be ok. I still feel that I have a long life ahead of me. I still feel like I will be here to help Ian grow up into an amazing man, to love and support Eric, to make my friends laugh, to simmer my mom and sister down, to paint for the world, to write a book...to laugh and love.

My power works best in weakness. – September 4, 2012

"My power works best in weakness." – 2 Corinthians 12:9

It is true. I never noticed the power, the strength, the grace of God more than when I feel weak, scared, lost... I don't know why, but it always amazes me when I do my daily devotional and when I read it, it seems like it was truly written just for me at the exact time I need it. In church Sunday, they sang a song that more than hit home, it touched my heart in a deep place. A place that used to not get touched much, but as this life continues a place that gets touched more often and because of it, I am a different person. The song went: I pray for you, you pray for me. And we watch God change things....

Yes I am scared. Yes the thought of the upcoming surgery freaks me out. Yes I want to wake up and realize this is a bad dream. Yes I am trying to control other things because this is so far out of my control. Yes I have been praying like a mad woman. Yes I believe all this will be ok. Yes I believe I will come out of this with flying colors, a cool new scar and a stronger heart. Yes it sucks...big time.

It has all really hit home today, the bigness of the whole situation. The appointments are made, people are on their way in to be with us...I feel like I am arranging my life from a faraway place. I still get waves of this floating sensation. It is a half dream/half-awake feeling then the reality of it all crashes into me and then I am fully awake with WTF is happening? How did this happen? When will this stop? And so much more. The next few days will be crazy. Please know that all your messages, emails, etc. are truly loved and welcomed even if I don't answer back.

Tomorrow 10:45am: meet with the neurosurgeon. After that go do pre-op check in and talk with the drug doctor (I can NOT for the life of me spell the correct word).

Thursday: 8:00am PET scan.

Friday: go into have brain surgery.

I have had a lot of people ask what we need. I don't know. I wish I knew, but I just don't know at this point. For now, please just pray for us. I will have Eric send an email on Friday.

This person I am... – September 6, 2012

I don't want to be brave

I don't want to be inspiring

I don't want to be strong

I don't want to have to be this person I have to be...

This person I am.

This person who doesn't have a choice

But to be strong

To be courageous

I want to breakdown

I want to say fuck it all

I want to eat my pain away

I want a magic wand to wave and all this shit to go away

Tomorrow is the day, brain surgery. I can't say I am not scared. I can't say I can make heads or tails out of this whole situation. I can't say I am ok.

Set me free and recuse me from the mighty waters – Psalm 144:7 – September 10, 2012

I am home from surgery and feel set free in a whole new way. I had so many quiet conversations with God while in the hospital recovering, holding His hand, leaning on Him for strength, and having full faith that even with this bump in the road, He has my back, He has bigger plans for me.

I really hope so.

I pray so, for bigger plans. I don't know if I could get through this if it were for nothing. Not nothing, I am getting through this for Eric and Ian. But I won't lie and not say that I hope there is more to the story. I guess I can't know if I stop reading?

Instead of me trying to figure out how to go about writing a book and getting it published I am going to just start writing, writing chapters, writing whispers to my heart, writing what I feel like He needs/wants me to say about all this. I am also excited to start painting more. I had vivid pictures in my mind about new paintings, new styles, and new ways to incorporate God's love into them to share with the world.

I will go see Dr. H this morning to set up brain radiation and according to her nurse, the talk with the medical director of BSI went very well on Friday. Please continue to pray that I get back on BSI and head radiation gets any last cancer straggler that might be hiding out. Thank you for all the prayers thus far and being with me in so many ways on this journey.

Where do I even begin? – September 30, 2012

To say the past 4 weeks have been hard, unnerving, life changing, healing and so much more is a huge understatement.

I got out of the hospital thinking, "oh, no big deal that I just had brain surgery" and why shouldn't I be able to just go on with life?

Well that "no big deal" caught up to me quickly and with a fierce force.

That following Monday after surgery, I had to jump right back into treatment and had zometa on top of it to boot. Then after treatment that day, my mom and I went to speak with the radiation oncologist. This meeting didn't go as I had expected. There was talk of whole brain radiation, half brain and possibly quarter brain. None of which I was expecting. I was expecting to radiate just the place that there was cancer, but I didn't realize the mass they cut out was about the size of a tennis ball.

I left there feeling defeated and scared.

Brain radiation freaks me out for many reasons and if all truth be told, I don't want to do it at all. I will do it because Eric has researched the heck out of it and it is better for me to do some sort of radiation versus nothing, but it still scares me and I still don't want to do it.

Tuesday and Wednesday I was able to rest with no appointments, which was great. All the information was still sinking in and the doom and gloom was starting to sink in too.

Thursday was treatment again. I still hadn't bounced back from zometa so I felt like I was kicked down again.

Friday, Eric and I went to speak with the CyberKnife doctor that my neuro doctor recommended.

Now here is the thing, I have been beyond blessed when it comes to doctors that I have. Their love and commitment to me is out of this world. So of course I was hoping to get the warm and fuzzies from this doctor. I didn't. He is very intelligent and has a great success rate at what he does, but his ability to talk to me in the words I need to hear...well, it wasn't happening. So we left there and I was even more confused and scared than when I went into this.

We went to eat at a local pizza place because it was after 1:30pm and I was starving. Then the pizza wasn't any good and I started to cry. Yes, I was crying in the middle of the pizza place. It really wasn't the pizza I was crying about. It was all this. I had been trying so hard to hold it all in, to hold it all together, to tell myself it would be ok when in fact I don't know shit and I am having a hard time believing anything I tell myself these days.

It sucks big time.

The weekend came and went. I hung out in bed a lot. I was still feeling "floaty" and out of my head. I could see my hands in front of me, but it took a lot to connect them to my thoughts. Weird I know. I feel like I am on a permanent high of some sort.

Monday was treatment again. Wednesday I went to see my neuro doctor to get 39 staples removed. Yes, 39 staples needed to come out of my head. It didn't hurt as much I thought it would, it was just uncomfortable. And after talking to him about the radiation, we decided to go with the CyberKnife. Thursday was treatment again.

Then we left on Sunday for Little Pink Houses of Hope retreat in North Carolina. Little Pink Houses of Hope is an amazing organization that provides FREE week long vacations for breast cancer patients and their families. They believe a cancer diagnosis does not just affect the patient, but the entire family. Every beach retreat is designed to help families relax, reconnect and rejuvenate during the cancer journey. The trip was great for Eric and Ian. Eric needed the calmness and serenity the beach brings him. Ian had a blast playing on the beach with Eric.

Hind sight now 20/20; that trip was not what I needed. I felt helpless that I wasn't able to help Eric with Ian, it took every ounce of energy I had to walk up and down the stairs to the condo and depression was starting to take root again. It came on faster and harder than ever before. There were a few times I thought to myself I wonder what would happen if I went swimming and never came back? How it would be hard for Eric and Ian at first, but it would have been better than this that they deal with on a daily basis.

It was hard for me to see other breast cancer patients there who felt great. And then I feel like an asshole even thinking that.

I had been that patient at one or more points in my life. The one who was going through treatment for the first time, or second or third and was able to keep that fucking smile on my face to show the world this cancer would not beat me, damn it!

Not now though. It was beating the life out of me.

Why should my not feeling good get to take away from them feeling great and having the times of their lives?

So, we didn't do much with the other families because I just couldn't. I couldn't keep that mask on and I didn't want to go out without it.

We are home now. And I must say I feel safe here at home. Treatment starts again tomorrow and hopefully I will figure out when/how long radiation will be. I guess I am now in the place of if I have to do this, let's do it and get it over with. It doesn't mean I am less scared or even want to do it, but I know I have to. All in all I am just "eh" about everything. I try hard not to put on a face of "oh it is alright" because in reality it isn't. It sucks. Only very few people will actually see my real face through this and for now I have accepted that. It is easier to put on the "oh it is alright face" but from that, I don't think anyone really knows how I hurt. I am not sure anyone really wants to know. It isn't fun, it isn't pretty and yes, it is very scary.

Normal...and such – October 15, 2012

I know I haven't written anything in a long time. I have Gina telling me all the time to write, to get it out there, to cleanse my mind all of which I know I need to do. I want to do but it has been hard. I went with Gina to pick up Ian today from school which was wonderful. I spent a lot of the day with her just hanging out like we used to.

I am not sure what my new normal will be or even how to get there. Some days I feel like normal is right around the corner, so close I could grab on to it and never let go. But the closer I get to it, the further it seems to slip away.

Other days I feel like no matter how hard I look, normal is nowhere in my line of sight.

It is funny though looking back reading about how I never wanted to be normal, to be someone who left something here on this earth, a trail of dust or something. Now, I pray to be normal. Someone with nothing special, just to live a normal life, with my normal family, in my normal house...just normal. I know this isn't going to happen, but I do wonder what it would be like...to be normal. Maybe normal is overrated?

I get radiation on my brain tomorrow...talk about not normal!

To be completely honest, I am scared of this, very scared. No one says there should be bad side effects, but come on, this is my brain we are talking about here. I will be mostly put out because I have to wear this mesh mask that pretty much locks my head to the table so I can't move.

While I was having the mask made, I starting getting a little antsy and freaked out because my head was screwed down to the table. I started thinking about Silence of the Lambs (NO idea why) and being as I was on the table for only half the time I will be on it tomorrow for the actual radiation treatment, the doctor said he will give me a little liquid cocktail to make it all easier. Hey, I am all for a little easier these days. I am done trying to prove I can do this on my own or without help. Please pray it all goes smoothly and really is a "normal" procedure.

I wish I knew...- November 1, 2012

I wish I could say sorry for not posting in such a long time, I can't though.

I haven't had it in me to write anything positive or write anything at all.

I wish I would have known what a complete toll this stupid brain surgery and radiation would have had on me.

I wish I would have known many things: How much more I should have appreciated feeling good when I did. How hard it is to feel bad. How it is all too easy to shut out the world but in reality that is the only thing I can do right at this moment. For those who are concerned with it, don't be. Don't take it personal, I am doing what I need to do for me and for my boys, that is all I can do right at this point.

I had to get another MRI on Monday because I was feeling like such crap over the weekend. The good news is there are no new areas of concern. The bad news is there is still a ton of swelling that was making me feel like crap. They upped my steroids, gave me new meds for the queasiness and I am praying for it all to start working….and soon.

I don't know how to reset from here. Some days are good, others aren't. I feel like when I am ready to hit the reset button and say this is it, this will be where my new normal starts, something happens and I start feeling worse again.

Prayers needed… - November 24, 2012

It has been a while since I have written. I am well aware of this. There is a good reason behind it.

A scary reason, the reality of my new life, reason.

I will start from the beginning of my last entry and lay it all on the line from there.

I ended up going to a different radiation doctor because I just didn't like the first one I went to. I felt like I was going to be a good "challenge" for him to add another notch to his belt loop. The one I ended up going with was great. He was kind and gentle and understood just how fragile I was at that time. He talked to me like a human and gave Eric his personal number in case we needed to get a hold of him at any time. AND he works closely with Dr. H and Dr. Cutie neurosurgeon. I had to get a metal-mesh-mask made again that will be screwed down to the table to hold my head in the exact place it needs to be all during radiation. I got the head radiation done and that was that.

But just like getting anything done to your brain, I was put back on steroids to help my newly radiated brain not swell. I don't know if radiation worked, but something was off from the get go. I knew it.

One afternoon a few days after radiation I had a big breakdown while on the phone with mom. My head had been hurting again, and I just had a feeling everything wasn't right. I keep telling mom I knew something was wrong and "it" was back.

I knew it was back. But in ALL the doctor's minds, there was no way the cancer could actually be back after the direct attack they just put the tumor through.

Not to mention they cut it out too.

Mom flew back to Austin to just stay with us for an undetermined amount of time.

The next two weeks, I pretty much stayed in bed and tried to numb myself any way I could. Be it with sleep, Xanax, or the many other pills I had to keep myself calm.

If I wasn't in bed, which was my protected place, I was pretty much having a panic attack. In those two weeks I had 2 MRIs to see what was going on because my head was killing me and I always felt sick to my stomach.

I kept having panic attacks thinking I felt another tumor growing. The MRIs kept showing something there, but everyone believed it was necrosis.

I didn't.

I believed I had another tumor in my head again.

With all this going on, I was at Dr. H's for a check-in appointment before chemo.

I couldn't do it anymore; I couldn't act like I wasn't crumbling, that I wasn't falling apart, that I wasn't scared for my life.

While waiting for Dr. H to come to my room, I crumbled.

I broke down, and I knew there was no putting me back together how things were.

Eric was there to hold my hand and calm me down. When Dr. H walked in and took one look at me, I could see the worry fill her eyes. She asked me a few things and all I remember was telling her I was just so tired, tired of it all and I just didn't know if I could go on.

She went and got her nurse to come stay with me while she talked to Eric in the hall. After that, I am not sure what happened next. I don't know if I blanked it out or what. According to Eric, Jennifer, Dr. H's nurse, came in to sit with me while Dr. H took Eric out into the hall way. I couldn't even walk out of her office down to our car. They had to wheel me down in a wheel chair for Eric to drive me over to the hospital. I honestly don't remember any of this. I remember mom somehow getting to the hospital after she took Ian to MDO and she stayed with me while Eric checked me it.

Not long after check in, I was admitted to a room. Dr. H and Eric decided I needed to be in there to rest, to not feel guilty about what was going on, and to watch me...there was a fear that I might try to hurt myself. I was in the hospital for four days trying to recover. I asked Eric and mom what was going on, and they told me I needed to rest. Dr. H put me in here to help me turn off my mind of daily stuff so I could rest.

Nothing made sense to me.

Between Eric and mom, someone was with me most of the time until it was time to get Ian and I would freak out again that no one was there to take care of him. Although, they assured me they had it all covered I couldn't let anything go.

I couldn't let any of it go.

My mind was in a constant state of panic that kept looping around again and again and again.

Dr. H would come visit me every day. The hospital therapist came to talk to me. I thought that was odd, but looking back at it now, I was in bad shape and they maybe thought I was going to try something, try something on myself; which in all honesty, I had thought about it. I thought about it a lot. I remember talking to the therapist though thinking, I can't tell him I have tried to stop breathing many times. I was starting to calm down and not think tumors were taking over my body.

But before they checked me out, they wanted one last MRI. Ok, no big deal. What was one more MRI at this point?

I got out of the hospital on Saturday and was starting to feel more like myself. I was able to function at least. I had BSI Monday, an appointment with Dr. Cutie neurosurgeon on Tuesday and BSI on Wednesday.

I wasn't real sure about the appointment with Dr. Cutie. I didn't remember it being on my calendar, but that didn't really mean anything concrete.

It hadn't been on my calendar.

From the MRI I had in the hospital, it was showing there was still a "mass" in the same spot that was changing. The neurosurgeon (Dr. Cutie) thought it was another tumor, the radiation oncologist thought it was necrosis from radiation (pretty much a big mass of dead cells that aren't going away) and Dr. H. just wanted to figure out what it was.

So with that, I was going back into surgery on Monday to have the mass removed.

My sister and her family came down for Thanksgiving dinner that my friends ordered in for us, and mom was still here to help which was a true Godsend.

I can say I was losing faith that it was going to be okay, but somehow I found peace with the upcoming surgery and felt that no matter what it is that is in there, once it is out all would be well again.

I had been having the same symptoms as before so I knew there was something in there.

Numb feet, slight headache and blurry vision on and off. Which could had be from necrosis or from something being in there. Now there was a slight chance the MRI on Monday before surgery will show the whole thing was gone and there wouldn't be surgery.

A reason?? – December 5, 2012

The pathology from the second mass removal came back and it showed it to be the same cancer as the first one (the same as the original breast cancer). I visited with Dr. H today and I left there feeling good. She said I am an odd case. Something none of them have seen before. But honestly I feel good about all this. I don't know why, but I feel good about it all. Odd I know, but I do feel like the brain stuff is gone. I felt all along since the first surgery that it wasn't done, but I feel different now. I go see a brain cancer doctor tomorrow. Yea, add another doctor to my list! <insert eye roll> I am not sure what to expect with him. I have a PET scan on Friday, and then treatment as usual (hopefully) will start back up next week.

So here is where I am: I truly trust I am going to be ok. I feel at peace with what has happened. I am not saying I have liked it or want to do it again, but I do feel like I will be ok. I will be healthy again. I will be here to raise Ian, to love Eric, to see my family and friends grow old. I am at peace with it all and I do feel like God has brought me through this for a reason...I am not sure what the reason is yet but there is a reason.

After getting home form surgery, it hit me hard...I might never be able to really walk by myself again. I was giving it about a week for the brain swelling to go down to start freaking out about my total numb right side...it has been a week. I am totally numb on my entire right side. I don't trust my legs to hold me up being as I can't feel them. Dr. H told me I needed to do in home PT. I am so done with all this shit at this point. I don't want to have to learn how to walk again. This isn't fair is all that swirls around my mind day in and day out.

I try to pray for this to be ok, but to tell you the truth, I am not sure God listens to me anymore. Really, how much can one person take? What else do I need to prove that I love Him and will spread

His love? I can't very well do any of that when I am having to heal all the time. I guess no one really cares about me telling them no. Mom has been here for every PT appointment and made me do it. She lets me cry and tell her I am tired, but she makes me do it. I think a thing only mom could make me do. I think God knew that and that is why he sent her again. That is what we do. PT in the mornings twice a week with Jason and PT on our own when he isn't there. Then I nap. Some days I feel like going to get Ian with mom from school, but some days I am just too tired and am afraid of getting motion sickness or a headache. I haven't really talked to many people lately. I don't have it in me to hold myself together and I feel like such a loser when I break down in front of others for no reason. Well no reason that is happening right there in that moment.

When I am with my friends I seem to just cry. It is too much for me, too much for my heart to handle. I cry for the way things used to be. I cry for how I wish things were. I cry because I can't walk without a walker or cane. I cry because Ian has to see me like this. I cry a lot. I had an appointment with Dr. Cutie to get my head stitches removed. After that was over, Eric asked me if I was up for Christmas shopping for Ian. We both knew I wasn't, but we both knew I so wanted to be a part of it. We went to Target, got me a battery operated cart and we were off. I drove and really tried not to hit people. It was nice to be out with Eric and laughing at this whole situation. We bought way too much, but I think I was buying because it made me feel like a better mom being as I feel like a horrible mom lately. I can't play with Ian, and if I tell the whole truth, I really don't want to. I don't know why. Well, yes I do. It reminds me of what I used to be able to do and what I am not able to do now. I told Eric the other night that I really feel like this might be my last Christmas. Of course he freaked out and told me I can't think like that. I just can't help it at this point. I really don't know what I have left in me. I feel like I have been put in the spin cycle

1189 times in the last 6 months and left out in the hot sun to finish the dry job.

Merry Christmas – December 25, 2012

We are at my sister's house and we all are a sight to see.

Me, well I have my walker and cane and can't stay awake for more than a few hours at a time.

My brother-in-law had major back surgery a few days ago. He can barely walk or stand up straight. So Shayne and I move from one couch, to the bed to watch TV and sleep while everyone does their thing.

Rachele is doing everything in her power to make this a great Christmas and I can't thank her enough. All the boys are playing and loving every second of it. Rachele, mom and Tammy are cooking way too much, but hey, that is what we do at the holidays.

I can't sit and chat with everyone for that long because laughing too hard makes my head hurt. I must say this is a good problem to have though...a very good problem indeed.

A Christmas miracle. Yesterday, all of a sudden I felt like I should try to walk with just my cane. I heard a little whisper in my heart that I could do it.

So I tried it.

And I did it!

I truly believe this is a Christmas miracle.

I am starting to taper off all of my steroids which is hard but good. I am still exhausted from recovering from the second surgery, PT and just mentally tired.

I am going to try to get my MRI on Thursday, so I can get my results on Monday the 31st. Please pray MRI is clear, treatment goes back to normal, and life (including driving) continues to get back to normal SOON!! I do feel God is guiding me through this, there is something bigger to this whole mess .I need to figure out what it is but it is coming. Thank you all for the love and support you have given to me, even if I haven't talked about it much, it means more than you will ever know. I love you all!

2013

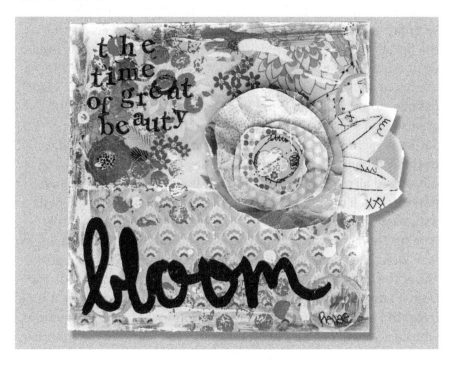

Happy New Year and more! – January 8, 2013

Things are FINALLY looking better around here. We had a
wonderful New Year's Eve. Eric grilled steaks, mom made potatoes,
Ian got to have a hot dog, we popped popcorn, watched a movie
and did a few fireworks out in the street. Ian was in a little slice
of heaven with the fireworks. It was so much fun to watch him
not have to have a care in the world except what was going on
right then and there. For all that, we were able to bargain with
Ian to sleep into 7:40am. Eric loved that since he is the awesome
one who always gets up with Ian being as sleep after treatment is
always great for me. Wednesday morning, mom, Ian and I were
able to meet Teri, Zach and Parker at Jungle Java for a play date.
It was so amazing to be able to get out and go do something with
Ian and friends again. I mean....SO AMAZING. I must say I am really
tired right now, but it was so worth it.

Friday we went over to Teri and Zach's to celebrate mom's birthday. It was a lot of fun too. Saturday I practiced driving for the first time since this whole brain thing happened and my leg went dead. I had to use my right foot for the gas and my left for the brake. I just didn't and still don't trust that my right foot can get over to the brake in time! But for my first spin out, it went great! Mom took me out yesterday and it went even better. Saturday night we took mom out to eat at Salt Lick for her real birthday dinner. Oh it was good! Sunday I was beat. I was in and out of bed all day napping on and off. It just really goes to show me how much my body is still recovering from everything. I had BSI (treatment drug) last Monday, Thursday, yesterday and this coming Thursday. I am still VERY swollen from the steroids. Like my face looks like I have gained probably 40 pounds. I was all worried about this at first, but now I am totally over it and what I look like. Even if I do keep on this steroid weight, I need to remember it is ok because I am alive. And who cares if I don't wear a size 8 anymore, who cares that I can't do what I used to. I can now do a lot more of different things. I am having my PT guy come over this morning to help me with my walking, then I plan on taking it easy until Ian gets home around 2:30pm.

So crazy to me... – January 23, 2013

This is still SUPER crazy to me...SUPER CRAZY. In May or June (HA...I can't remember!) of 2011, my sweet neighbor Holly asked me if she could take pictures of me and my bald head...I said sure. When she gave me the pictures, she had me sign a release...I had no idea what for. Then back in August or September (again, can't remember exact details!) she briefly told me my pictures were a hit. She might have told me more details, I might have asked more, but I don't remember. Then the other day I was outside and she came over to chat and for a hug and she told me again about my pictures and since I am more with it, I asked a little more. Then she brought us veggie chili a few days later and I asked her more about the pictures and I told her that Eric's parents had been telling us they could swear a picture of me was on a billboard on the way "up North" to their lake house.

I really had NO IDEA what they were talking about...I kept telling Eric I was NOT on a billboard. But after talking to Holly, she told me that yes I probably was on a bill board because she put my pictures on a site where people purchase pictures. And I guess cancer companies liked my pictures...here are some links (if I can remember how to post links...you think I am kidding?)

Fred Hutchinson Research Center donation page - https://www.fhcrc.org/en/how-to-help.html

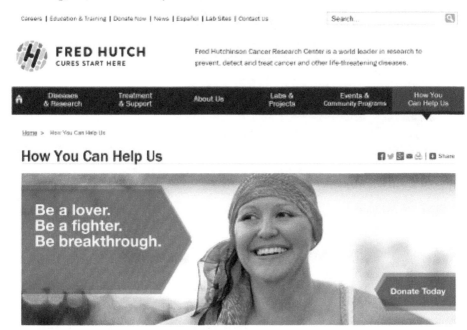

I have billboard pictures too (one from MI, Eric's parents, and one

from Seattle, a pink ribbon cowgirl spotted it while in Seattle) but I can NOT for the life of me figure out how to post a picture from a file...it is times like these that I remember I had 2 brain surgeries and radiation within a 90 day period...when my brain doesn't work.

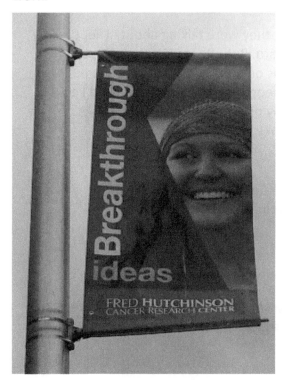

And now I am even International!

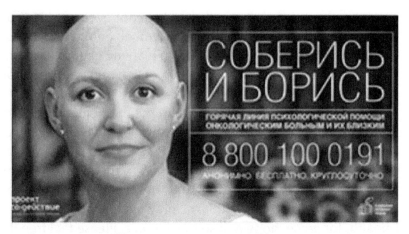

СОБЕРИСЬ
И БОРИСЬ

ГОРЯЧАЯ ЛИНИЯ ПСИХОЛОГИЧЕСКОЙ ПОМОЩИ
ОНКОЛОГИЧЕСКИМ БОЛЬНЫМ И ИХ БЛИЗКИМ

8 800 100 0191

АНОНИМНО БЕСПЛАТНО КРУГЛОСУТОЧНО

7 лет работы и 55 тысяч
абонентов - сегодня у нас...

us7.campaign-archive1.com

My take on The Spoon Theory – January 30, 2013

Eric told me about this article he read called The Spoon Theory written by Christine Miserandino. She has lupus and she writes a blog called But You Don't Look Sick. The title of the blog really hit home with me. I know many other stage IV women, who when you first look at them you would never think that they have stage IV cancer...heck before this whole brain mess, I was one of those while I was on the parp. I now feel like I look sick...with my foot issue and the big scar and bald spot on the back of my head...you know, it is the little things. It really hit home with me because I have been having a hard time lately with my lack of energy and I always feel on the defense with others when I say I can't do something. I mean, I look like I should feel fine, I look so much better than I did even a few a weeks ago, I am able to walk without a cane, so I should be back up and running...right??

I am nowhere near full speed...hell I am not even near 25% of full speed most days. Everything takes so much energy...takes a spoon or two or three from my pile. I try to plan my days to have enough spoons left to share some with Ian and Eric...some days it works, some days it doesn't. And the hardest part is that I never know what the day will be like until I am in the moment. Some days I wake feeling great and then crash, other days I feel good all day, still others I wake up tired, my foot is heavy and it is hard to move. I am trying to be ok with this. Some days I am ok with it, some days I'm not...I want more...more energy, more ability to walk, more feeling in my foot...all the things I pray for. I pray for patience, for health, for grace, hope and so much more. Please feel free to pray with me. I have really found that when I ask for specific prayers from y'all, God works in even more amazing ways. Please pray for complete feeling to return to my right foot, to stay cancer free in my whole body today, tomorrow and always and love to always pour out of me.

Explanation: - February 12, 2013

I have been thinking about this for a long time. I have a lot to say, but it is hard to find the words, even to write the words. I finally feel like I am in a place to talk about things, to explain myself, to all those I have shut out this entire time...maybe?? I just couldn't talk about it before. I still can't talk about it in person, I don't really know why. It is still so fresh...I am still so scared...so many untouched emotions. I watched a Criminal Minds episode last night that was recorded from a while ago. I don't usually watch this show because it is a little too much for me, but it was a follow up to one that was dealing with one of the main characters losing a loved one. This episode showed him blocking out his friends and family and it really hit home with me. I completely understood it, he knew they were there for him, but he just couldn't deal with the emotions talking about it would bring. I know no one has asked for an explanation, but I need you to know...Me shutting everyone out wasn't what I wanted to do, it was all I knew to do...it was all I could do. I couldn't talk about what I had been through...what we were still going through, it was too much for me to wrap my head around. But then on the other hand I couldn't go on with "normal" life because my world, my life, my everything had been more than flipped upside down. I didn't know if I was going to survive it all, I didn't know if Ian was going to have a mom to help raise him, I didn't know if Eric was going to have a wife.

I didn't know anything. I didn't want pity but at the same time I wanted people to realize how bad it sucked. Yes, I realize people can't know how bad, how hard it was because I didn't tell them...I am still working on that. There was a lot that went unsaid. I had no energy to do anything other than survive. I had no energy to talk to people, to write here or write back to people, to be alive, all I could focus on was making it through to the next day, heck, even through to the next minute. Surviving took it all, every ounce of anything I had. I still don't know what I need from others. I try to think about what I would do for others if the situation was reversed and I realize I don't know what I would do. I would want to ask them what they need and so many asked/still ask what we need. I still don't know what to say. I guess I need love and understanding. I know I have both of these from so many people and I know it is hard to continue to give love without getting any in return from me...but that is what I need now. What I want to say when asked this is *I need new cells...cells that don't want to divide on their own and cause cancer.* I need new DNA (I really don't know if this is DNA stuff), what I need is stuff no one can give me. So do I tell people this when they ask? I don't, it doesn't do anyone any good for me to be a smartass all the time...some of the time yes! I still haven't really explained anything here, I realize that. I guess I still don't know how to explain it; I am not sure I will ever know how to explain what I went through and continue to go through every day. But please know your love and support does not go unnoticed and it does make things so much easier, if I don't tell you that enough, it is true.

On our own – February 17, 2013

Eric's mom and dad left Saturday morning. This is the first time we are "on our own" since October 22nd, that was when my mom came back because I was convinced something wasn't right. Mom had been here through the end of January, and then his parents got here a day after she left. They were willing and able to stay longer, but about twelve days ago, things started changing again... huge changes...miracles happening right before our eyes.

My energy wasn't just creeping back, but it seemed to come back in a huge burst AND it has stayed. I even had zometa on Monday and it didn't knock me down.

I have been practicing driving for the past month, and I feel comfortable driving a few places, so I started going a few places: I started taking and picking up Ian by myself, I went over to Gina's for lunch, I met Sylvia at the park one day and Jungle Java another day. Things are truly falling into place. So, his parents witnessed all these magnificent things taking place and asked if we were ready to be on our own. We talked about it, and we were, so now we are.

40 shades of grey – February 22, 2013

And no, this has nothing to do with the book out there...believe me I only wish it was that simple. I got my MRI results yesterday from the MRI on Wednesday. The gist of it is: there has been a change to the surgery bed, BUT more than likely it is my brain healing. My neuro oncologist (Groves) told Dr. H he wants to go to four week MRIs versus six weeks...just to keep a closer eye on it all...which is fine with me. I talked to Dr. H's nurse when she gave me the report but now I have more questions AND I lost the report so I need to have her email it to me. I go see the radiation doctor (Shinebine)on Tuesday, so I am guessing we will have more info then. Yes, Eric is going with me so he will remember the conversation! I can really see how Ian wants a black or white answer from me when he asks me something, this living in the grey zone is hard. I am trying to get used to it and know there is no black or white answer.

Now versus then... – March 5, 2013

Eric and I were talking about where I am now versus three months ago right after the second surgery, wow, what a difference.

Since the second surgery (calling it a brain surgery and the thought of my head being cut open and parts of my brain being cut out still really freaks me out...really) my life has, our lives have changed multiple times.

I think what has happened isn't even called change.

I don't know what it is called...maybe we are just continuing to grow and accept it all and just let it flow.

I have gone from using a walker to a cane to walking on my own! I continue to pray that the full feeling comes back to my right side again. I was never grateful enough for both legs and feet having full feeling...it was one of those things I never thought I would lose. I assumed it was there, now and forever. I am now working on walking in crowds. The stop, go, dodge, step side to side really throws me. I get nervous, flustered with myself and the surroundings, I am afraid of falling. It is like I am learning to walk all over again. Well quite honestly I am. But this time around I am much higher off the ground and a fall would hurt much worse...and I am well aware of it. I guess it is a good thing that we are so young and "bounce able" when we learn to walk.

I saw Dr. H yesterday, I love seeing her. We went over my last MRI and she said it isn't as grey as I had thought. She talked to the "team" she confers with on my case...it still seems to intrigue them and they all love seeing the MRI results. The results: yes there is still grey matter (well beside my brain) and the spot where the cancer was is still different from the rest of my brain but it looks more like scar tissue now. She showed us this MRI versus one in Dec and it is amazing how different it looks. It is like the brain that was removed and the scar tissue filling in the "hole" is molding to my brain and just forming around it. Seeing all this makes my belief in God that much more, I mean the thought of these amazing things taking place, my brain knowing what to do to heal itself. It is a miracle and so amazing to even think about. This is where everyone thought I was going to be soon after the first go around... well, we all know how that turned out!! I am feeling more and more like myself daily and I thank God all the time for it.

Test results – March 23, 2013

My adventures in Cancerland continue. As someone suggested the first time I wrote about Cancerland, she envisioned a board game like Candy Land, but in my case it is Cancerland. Sometimes you move forward, sometimes you move back, sometimes you get stuck... It has been an up and down week around here, and the rollercoaster will continue into next week...I really, REALLY just want a week that is flat. Flat with no excitement, flat with no worry, flat....flat...flat...FLAT! I would be extremely happy to even move just one place forward. This week I moved 3 forward and 5 back...or so I feel like and now I'm stuck in goo and wait my turn. MRI results look great!! The cavity is filling in and there is NO GROWTH (that is all I ever want to hear!) PET scan, all looks great, BUT one area on my pancreas that is there now and hasn't been before. But the deal is, there are only like 11 reported people that have had breast cancer move to the pancreas, so EXTREMELY RARE, but in my case, my body seems to like the rare stuff. The long and short of it is, I will get a CT with contrast then will know more. I have it in my head whatever was showing up was from acupuncture on Thursday that got my chi moving and the pancreas is a big part of that process! Regardless, I am asking for prayers, that the "interesting spot" is miraculously gone and there is nothing to ever look at. I will keep y'all posted with more adventures of Renee in Cancerland.

Ripples in the water – April 3, 2013

What I didn't realize was that my sickness, my illness, my cancer... whatever you want to call it is like a rock being thrown into a calm still lake. A lake so still it is like glass, so still you can see your reflection. My little part of the greater lake has been disturbed; a rock has been thrown in the middle making ripples that continue making other ripples. Though the ripples aren't contained only to the spot where the rock broke through the water. I am seeing now that my cancer is like a rock being thrown into the lake, the lake we are all a part of, the lake where all of our lives mold together... sway back and forth with the water...the pulse of life. What I didn't understand, or didn't see is that my ripples reach out way beyond what I can see...all of our ripples do. The ripples of each of our lives can affect so much...for miles and miles out. The ripples can shake the fish swimming, they can move the sand under our feet, they can sway the reeds that usually stand up so straight and tall... the small tiny ripples can and do affect so much more than I could ever imagine. I am seeing how my ripples are affecting those that

I love in so many different ways, ways I don't know how to talk about, ways that break my heart, ways that make me angry, ways that can change lives.

The ripples, the after effects of my cancer ripping into my brain, the effect of the fact settling in on most everyone...just what Stage IV cancer can do, the ripples are forever changing my shoreline, my life line to others...and forever changing those around me, those who love me...my ripples are forever changing their shorelines too. The ripples are all different: different sizes, different strengths, effect different parts of the shoreline. Some are large ripples that turn into waves, waves that change everything in its path as soon as it hits. Some are oh so gentle, so gentle you barely even notice they are there, changing the landscape around you. These ripples I speak of now were first caused by me having Stage IV breast cancer, non-curable cancer, Stage IV...just the word itself was the rock that was thrown into my smooth, beautiful lake.

These ripples slowly started creating new ripples. Now I feel like my life has been taken over by ripples instead of the nice smooth water that once was. I have learned that all ripples are created by something by some sort of something breaking the surface of each person's own lake. Some ripples are caused by fear, fear of me dying. How much time does she have here on earth...with me? Some ripples are caused by anger, anger at God or whoever has let this happen. How could He let this happen to a mom, a wife, a sister, a friend, a daughter? Some ripples are caused by shame, what if someone did something to cause this. What if I did this to me? What if I ate something bad one too many times? Some ripples are caused by thanksgiving, thanksgiving that I am still alive. Thank God, I am still here to love and be loved. Some ripples are caused by joy, joy of every day. Joy for the simple things, the sitting quietly in the togetherness of friendship and family. Some ripples are overshadowed by darkness, darkness of the unknown. What if the cancer comes back? Some ripples are caused by sorrow. What do I not get to experience because of cancer? All these ripples float in my lake daily....in and out, never stopping.

I am now learning that these ripples ripple through the lakes of my loved ones too...they always have even without cancer. All of our ripples ripple through each other's lakes. Sometimes we try to stop the ripples from coming into our lake, but to do that we must put up a wall, a wall that blocks out more than just the ripples. Some lakes have all the ripples my lake has, some lakes only have the dark and scary ripples that seem to tear the water's surface daily, some lakes try to get rid of the ripples by stopping all the motion which actually only make the ripples worse. I am learning to accept the ripples to let them come and go as they please, to let them change my shore as they need but I am to the point where I will no longer fight with my ripples, it is a losing battle and I have found out if I sway with the ripples, they are actually quite pleasant.

Good news...GREAT news – April 5, 2013

Got the call today, the biopsy came back from my GI scope on Monday....wait for it....wait for it...NO CANCER!! It is just an ulcer; I never thought I would say *just an ulcer*. I think it is from all those damn steroids, they can cause major stomach acid. Whatever, not cancer is all I wanted to hear!

Firsts...again – April 9, 2013

Getting back to what I was able to do before the brain tumor has been one blessing after another. Yesterday was a big day for me

- used to be a normal day. I read somewhere that everything we do should be celebrated; therefore, we should be thankful for everything, even the tiny things that seem like no brainers, things we assume will never go away. I now realize there is nothing we can assume…as we don't know anything for sure.

I went on a 20 minute walk around the park after I dropped Ian off. The "old me" would look at that and roll my eyes. I took Ian to Michael's craft store for the first time since last August, before this I couldn't go alone; just the thought of the store overwhelmed me…in all aspects.

In the past four months: I have walked with a walker, then with a cane, then with a brace and am now walking on my own.

I relearned to drive and made it to the Grocery store with just me and Ian.

I can now do laundry; I can't carry the baskets because it throws my balance off. I can load and unload the dishwasher. We went to the mall. Again, all this stuff I used to do without once thinking these were huge blessing. Now, I say thank you all day long for what I can do again.

Layers – April 13, 2013

I am starting to see my life

All life, as I see my paintings

Layers upon layers

Some layers are one color

Some layers add texture

Some layers are every different color of the rainbow

Some layers turn out like mud

Some layers are flat and shiny

Some layers are rough around the edges because I tried to sand something off that I thought Shouldn't be there

Though- I see now even the ugliest layers

Even the ones I thought were pure beauty

Don't matter when looked at alone

They all only matter when looked at as a whole picture

And I see now that even when I think

I am done adding layers

There is always room for more

More texture, more colors, more love

Layers in Pictures

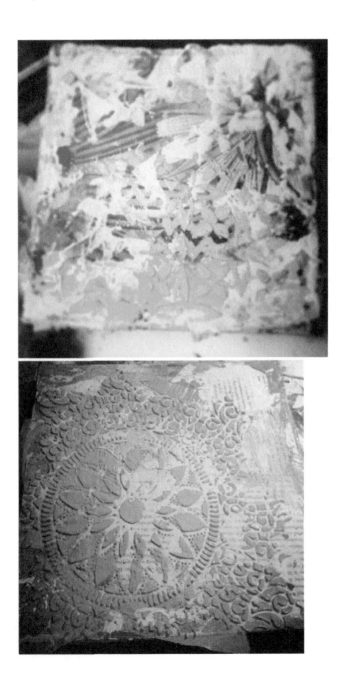

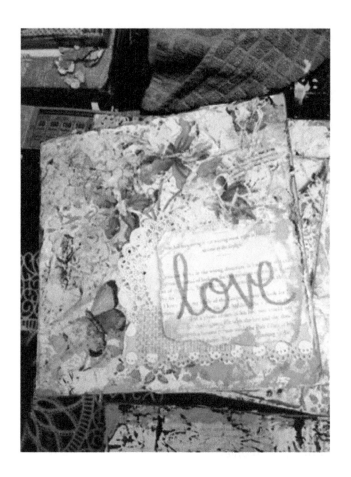

How do I still believe? – April 15, 2013

She asked me how,

how could I still believe in God...

in a loving God?

How could I still believe?

Because she couldn't,

she couldn't believe after this,

after me.

After me having Stage IV cancer at 32 years old...

Stage IV non-curable cancer.

How did I still believe?

When I got cancer when I was 30,

 when my only child was 13 months old?

Cancer in my brain?

How did I still believe God was good?

My question to her was,

how do you not believe God is good?

Do you not see the love that surrounds me?

The pure love from my family and friends, that love is from God.

The love from Eric that never waivers.

The love from my doctors and nurses who take care of me.

God gives that love to us all, fills our hearts with love to share it all the time with those who need it.

Do you not see the grace He gives me?

The grace to smile day to day, even if it is always in the back of my mind, what if "it" comes back?

The grace to tell the truth about it all, even in my darkest hours.

The grace to cowgirl up because I have to do what I have to do, even when going to treatment for the second time every week is the last thing I want to do.

Do you not see that grace?

God gives me that grace.

Do you not see the miracles that happen before our eyes?

Me getting on my trial drug one week, ONE WEEK before it closed.

Me having the courage to insist I knew something was wrong after my first brain surgery, to pretty much tell my doctors they were wrong and the tumor was back even though it wasn't showing up on scans.

Me walking again.

Me being alive to continue to love.

These are all miracles, big and small from Him.

These are all just the tip of the iceberg of my list of miracles.

But you can't see Him, how do you know? She pressed on.

You can't see the wind but you can feel it on your skin.

You can't see love but you feel it when you hold your child.

You can't see hurt but you feel it when your heart breaks.

You are right you can't see Him, but you see signs of Him everywhere you look.

Yes, I believe.

Yes, I know God is good and God is love.

Learning to listen – April 18, 2013

It is hard for me to remember that I had two brain surgeries (well, Eric says 3 because radiation is counts as a surgery) a little over 6 months ago. It is hard for me to remember that my body needs time...needs time to rest more than most, time to recover, just time.

It is hard for me to remember that I receive chemo twice a week.

It is hard for me to remember that if I push too hard one week, it takes me a lot longer to bounce back the next.

It is hard for me to remember because it all seems so normal to me. I pushed too hard last week on my off week...and I am still trying to bounce back this week.

I crammed too much into my week, too many appointments, too many errands, too many lunch dates, which so sucks to say that because I crave those lunch dates, I crave that time with my friends. I haven't yet been able to find a balance on my off weeks...I always do too much of something and then the bounce back is slow, then I beat myself up and then, well, you know the rest of the cycle. I am praying I learn my boundaries and when I can push them and when I need to accept them and surrender to them. I am praying I learn to listen to my body and its needs.

WALK FOR RENEE – April 21, 2013

My best friends from the neighborhood girls decided they had had enough of me not letting them help me. They put together "Walk for Renee". It was a Halloween in April theme, because who doesn't like dressing up?!

The outpouring of love was magical, you could see the glow of love all around, the air seemed charged with love.

The support was beyond belief. The fun had by all was fantastic. The smiles on all the faces showed the enjoyment I felt in my heart. It was an amazing day.

To those who were there, I hope you all had the amazing time I had. I hope you all enjoyed all the smiles and heart felt love I was able to enjoy., I know my thank you doesn't even touch the tip of the gratitude I have for all the work put into this, for all the people who were there and all the people who wanted to be there. I am more than blessed with y'all in my corner cheering me on and your continued prayers. I love you.

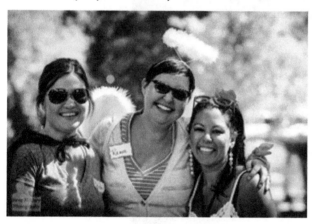

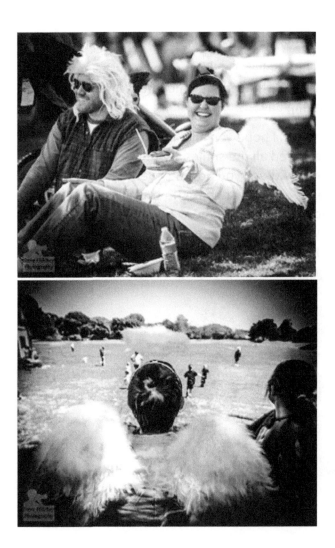

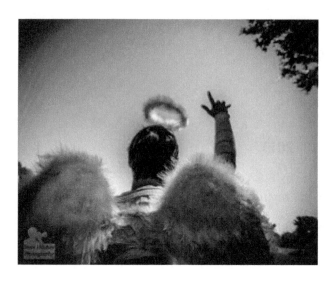

I believe – April 25, 2013

I believe God lives inside

Inside us all...

After all – He did make us all

I believe He made Himself a warm loving home in all our hearts

I believe God is always talking

To guide and love us

And our hearts... our hearts can only hold

So much so much love

Before it overflows like a cup too full of liquid

So, you see there is no choice

But to let that Love

Overflow

Overflow onto us all

From us all

Bag lady – April 28, 2013

I have collected bags all my life

As long as I can remember

Some big

Some small

Some stylish

Some plain

These bags –

These bags I collect

Even hoard

These bags hold all

Different kinds of

Emotions

Stories

Hurts

Loves

Dreams

Failures

Hopes

Lately though

I have realized

These bags

All weigh different

Love is light and airy

I can sling it over my shoulder and take it with me wherever I go –

No matter how long the journey

Joy is the same

I can stuff my bag full of joy

And never feel its weight on my shoulder

Thought-

On the other hand

Anger

Shame

Hate

Guilt

Can weigh me down

Even if I am only carrying

A single

Lonely

Pebble in my bag

This tiny pebble

Weighs a ton

Like I am carrying bricks

Bending me

Side to side

Hurting my body

Little

By

Little

Tweaking my back

Here and there

I have decided though

I surely don't need

All these bags

Weighing me down.

I am getting rid of the bags

Especially the tiny bags

The tiny bags

That carry only the pebbles

The pebbles

That weigh me down

Instead

I only need one bag

One bag

To carry God

With me all day everyday

In that bag

I will find

All the

Love

Joy

Grace

Laughter

Hope

I can imagine

And this,

This bag for God

Will be the only bag

I carry from now on

Hold my hand – May 15, 2013

I am not sure where to even start or where to even go with this – with this whole situation I am once again facing.

The rug has once again been yanked out from under my feet. At this point, I feel like I have a mean gremlin following me around just to mess with me.

I want to be strong but I feel like my courage it seeping out faster than God can refill my cup.

I want to understand but I know I never will. So then I try to give it away – all of it away to God, but let me tell you friends that is hard. There always seems to be a tiny piece that latches on and lingers.

Let me back up a few days.

After leaving chemo treatment, I went to have lunch – yes, I go eat by myself after treatment on a regular basis...yes, all those people there know me too!

I was walking out from the restaurant to my car, and I felt it...I felt my leg go number.

I know this is hard to comprehend, but I am used to the normal numbness of my right leg. It is when it gets heavier than my normal and my shoulder area goes numb too is when I hit the panic button.

I got in my car, called Jennifer at Dr. H and told her something was wrong...she knew how serious I was because I was crying. I can usually hold it together until I have something to cry about...I knew I had something to be crying about.

As usual, they worked their magic and got me in for an MRI that day.

Eric came home to drive me, Ian went to a friend's house, and I was wrecked – wrecked with fear, anger, sadness – you name it and I am sure it went through me.

We got a call early the next day from Dr. Cutie's office asking us to come in that afternoon.

Eric and I walked in not at all ready for what was there.

Dr. Cutie had my MRI pictures up. As soon as we walked into the where he was, with my MRI on the computers – I took one look at the images, at his face and cried.

It is back...the mother fucking brain tumor is back in the same spot.

I looked at him dumbfounded. I wanted to ask how, but he beat me to it. He told me he had never seen anything like this before, and he wished he knew how...

Then there we were again – deciding when to do my 3rd brain surgery in 10 months.

I told him that I get it, it had to be done, but I also told Dr. Cutie that I just want to be able to walk after this surgery – and I am fine even if that is with a cane.

That is when they broke - the strong men broke. Eric and Dr. Cutie had tears leaking out of their eyes.

I told them if I have to choose one – walk or use of my right hand – I will take the use of my hand to draw, paint and write.

More tears were shed.

I told them that I don't think it is fair for me to think if I have to choose one.

Oh Sweet Sweet God – please heal me, please protect me, please be with me through this all and carry me to the other side of the valley

I am scared

So do not fear, for I am with you; do not be dismayed, for I am your God. I will strengthen you and help you; I will uphold you with my righteous right hand. Isiah 41:10

Surgery is scheduled for first thing Thursday morning.

I am going to a Prayer Warrior today after dropping Ian off at school, then my mom and sister will be here and hopefully we will get pedicures at some point today?

Please pray first and foremost this is just necrosis – that means just scar tissue and no tumor.

Please pray for God to guide all my Doctors and comfort my family and friends.

Update – May 20, 2013

Ok, ok, ok. I don't want to say it too soon but third time might actually be the charm!?!?

I was released from the hospital after only a one night stay. Dr. Cutie said yes it is odd to release me a day after brain surgery, but he knows me well enough to know I will call if I need something.

My right foot feels like I am wearing a cast boot on my foot and my leg/foot is still super heavy BUT I CAN WALK!! It is slow and awkward, but I can do it! Thank you all for all the prayers, love and more prayers. I see my radiation doctor this week, and then we will go from there.

Check in – May 25, 2013

I know some of you are curious to see how your prayers have been heard!

Let me list the ways! This past week has been really good. Ian graduated "advanced pre-k" on Tuesday. It was so sweet, and yes, of course I cried.

I had an appointment with my brain radiation doctor yesterday. All is well. I get a mask sometime next week and we are going to do a higher but smaller area doses of radiation. I will more than likely have three to five treatments. My radiation doctor is getting with my brain surgeon to see if he wants to come be a part of this process too. I mean really?! REALLY??? I know I am more than TRULY blessed with my doctors, but they are so above and beyond in every way I could ever imagine. Pretty much like God just put them here to help us out!

Next week will be a busy week again. Dr. H is still not sure on my trial drug situation. Eric and I have talked, and we are leaving it in God's hands. If they kick me off the trial, and I need to be on a new one, then so be it. On May 29th, I will get my radiation mask made. Party time for me!! I get good drugs while they create a mold of my face to hold my face in place. I am going to take videos this time to document it. The final time! On May 30th, I will have another MRI. On June 3rd, I see Dr. Groves. I am not sure what will be happening at this one. In between all this, we are packing up our house and getting ready to move!!

It is official...I have been kicked off my trial drug – May 29, 2013

I am kind of in shock, kind of not, kind of ok, and kind of not ok???

I was officially kicked off my BSI trail drug yesterday.

I feel a few things here but am still wrapping my head around this.

On one hand I am scared. I feel like BSI has kept my "body" clean since I started it in September, 2011. I say "body" because my brain is not included with this. The BSI has never been able to cross the blood brain barrier. BSI effects are known to me. I knew I would get it every Monday and Thursday. That was my job. I would go to treatment 2 times a week. I had my routine. I knew when I would and wouldn't feel good and I knew the BSI was working.

On the other hand, I was/am ready for a change on many levels. I was tired of going twice a week. I was tired of being tired. But now I realize that that tired might be NOTHING compared to what my new tired might be. Only time will tell. I was tired of being tied to that schedule but now I am thinking what in the hell am I going to do without that schedule?

I was tired of not being able to go out of town for longer periods of time. But I knew, I knew what I was going to feel like. I do feel in my heart it will be good, but that doesn't mean I am not scared of the unknown.

My schedule for the next two weeks are a little crazy, but we have come to realize this is life and just like every life all we can do is live in the moment we are in.

May 29th: I go get fitted with my radiation mask.

May 31st: I get my head stitches out. I can't believe it has only been two weeks since my third brain surgery.

June 3rd: Ian starts karate camp. I think it's going to be GREAT fun for him!

June 6th: I see my brain chemo doctor to see what the plan is.

June 7th: I see Dr. H and sometime within all of the above, I will be getting radiation again. I should find that out today what that schedule is.

Jeremiah 29:11 - Holding tight to His plan – June 4, 2013

"For I know the plans I have for you, declares the LORD, plans to prosper you and not to harm you, plans to give you hope and a future." – Jeremiah 29:11

I am holding tight to this verse, OH so tight. I know He has plans and as hard as it is to admit it to myself, I don't know the plans and I shouldn't know the plans ahead of time. I just need to know He has a plan and is putting it into place this second. There has been a slight change of plans this week. After my radiation doctor and my neurologist spoke, they came up with a new plan. I will do brain radiation on Wednesday, Thursday and Friday versus just one day. I will go in at 4:30pm daily to get the good drugs to relax me, being as I will have to be strapped to the table with a mesh face mask. (Yes, I have pictures.) Radiation will be 5:00pm to5:30ish. As much as I do NOT want to do three days of radiation on my brain, I do trust this plan but I am scared. I am scared of so much right now. I am tired of being scared. I know one could say if I am scared I don't truly trust His plan, and that could be the case. I really don't know at this point. One day of radiation seemed to totally throw me over the edge last time into crazy town and zapped every last ounce of energy I had left. And I still don't know what "maintenance" I will be on. I am ready for a plan. I guess looking back my Monday/Thursday plan wasn't so bad. I actually miss going there twice a week. I kind of feel like I have lost a group of friends and now will be an outsider.

Brain radiation starts today: - June 5, 2013

I am getting nervous about the radiation that will start today. It seemed radiation was what threw me over to crazy town last time, but I think I have a better handle on it this time, but I don't know. And really, I don't think radiation is what threw me over to crazy town. I think I had been balancing on the edge for some time and that was the gust of wind that blew me over. I guess I won't know until after it is over though? I feel myself getting nervous. I am trying to line things up around the house, make sure Ian has something to do this weekend because I know I am going to need to "just be" most of weekend and for that I already feel guilty. I know I will need to be alone, it to be quiet, just be able to heal. There is way too much nervous energy around here.

Mom and I are going to go get me a new purse and then go out to lunch while Ian is at camp before Eric takes me to radiation. I guess I shouldn't have a glass of wine at lunch before my brain gets blasted with radiation?!?!

Radiation pictures, day 2 and brain chemo doctor today – June 6, 2013

Yesterday ended up being a great day. I decided that although I was tired and lying on the couch sounded great, it would be better for me to get out and about a bit before radiation started. Mom and I went shopping. I got two cute fedora style hats to wear because I am pretty sure I will have a bald spot again and Austin sun plus bald spot equals no good. Then home for a bit to nap. Mom went and got Ian from camp and then took him on a date for ice cream and the pool. What a great BB he has! I don't know how we would do this without her here. Then Eric and I went to radiation. It took longer than I expected, but they were being VERY precise. I will take that! I really don't want more radiation than I need. I can just imagine my brain blowing up from it. Here is the machine I am in. Yes I am strapped down with all those layers of mesh to ensure I don't move my at ALL. I did ok until about half way through then I had to request a second dose of anxiety medicine because I was starting to freak out from the pressure of the mask that was giving me a HUGE headache. Today I go see Dr. G - my brain oncologist in the morning 2nd radiation treatment this afternoon Please pray radiation goes smooth today and my doctors have a plan for me tomorrow.

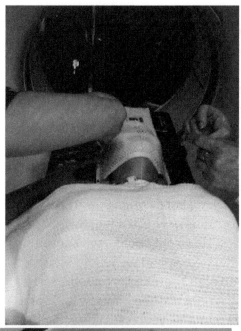

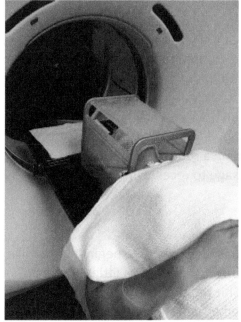

Brain oncologist and day 2 of radiation – June 7, 2013

I went to see Dr. Groves yesterday. If I haven't said it enough, let me say it more, I am so beyond blessed with the team of doctors I have working with me and with each other it amazing me. Completely amazes me. So Dr. Groves thinks I am an interesting case. I told him I like to be interesting, and he said he likes my attitude! I think we will make good partners! Our plan from his end is to send in every last bit of cancer tissue they have from me and all my previous surgeries' to get it all reanalyzed for more of a genotype. They have been doing this from each surgery but he is going to go as in depth as possible, something like 200 mutations to look for. I told him even though it keeps coming up triple negative (i.e., not caused by hormones), I have a feeling it has something to do with hormones. He said it could have something to do with hormones like five tiers down and we would figure it out...very exciting stuff! Eric and I left there feeling good even though we didn't have a plan. I go back to see him July 11th for a plan. (After our trip up to Eric's parents...yeah vacation!!)

After that appointment, I was so tired but these stupid steroids give me this nervous energy. I can't focus or sit still even though I am exhausted. Eric got here at 4:00pm to take me to radiation. While we were on the way to radiation, the radiation nurse called and said their machine shut off and was warming back up so they were now running about an hour and half late. No biggie, we did an early dinner. We stopped by REI to get Eric a hat for Father's Day and ended up finding a rubber boomerang for Ian. I am making him a little fun package to receive in the mail. He loves getting mail...who doesn't?!?!

Off to radiation: They gave me my cocktail in the beginning just like yesterday and about half way through gave me a little more pain medication due to the mask. It hit the pressure point right across my forehead and it really started to hurt and freak me about after a bit. But, I made it and all is well. We got home to quiet because mom and Ian were out with Syl and her family. Mom is taking Ian to Fort Worth this weekend which is hard for me to say, but that makes me happy. I feel like the peace and quiet is going to be the best thing for me at this point. It was hard to tell them I need them to go away for the weekend, but Ian couldn't be more excited to so see the boys and mom enjoys the trip too!

Day 3 radiation down and a bit of a plan – June 8, 2013

I visited with Dr. H yesterday. Yes I was feeling lost without having seen her for a little over a week or even being there at her office. Between her and Dr. Groves, we are all on the same page, sending any and all tissue we have out for mega proto typing.

July 8th: I will have another MRI.

July 11th: I will go to Dr. Groves.   And on

July 17th: I will go back to see Dr. H.

In between all of this, I am going to rest and recoup from surgery and brain radiation.

I am still not able to sleep through the night. I am not sure why so I am feeling like a walking zombie most of the time.

Mom is still here helping with Ian. My friends are still keeping us fed. I am going to try to paint today. I feel the need to get out all the emotions that have settled in my heart, and painting just seems to let it flow like nothing else.

Please keep praying His hands are guiding any and every decision made, Eric and I have handed it all over.

What is breast cancer to me? – June 12, 2013

I have been thinking about this topic for a LONG time now, but it is hard to put into words. I have a lot more to say, but I have to process it, so I will write it as it comes. What is breast cancer to me? It is a lot more than the pretty pink ribbons people like to doll it up with. Well, some people. Cancer, any cancer is not pretty. Cancer is hard. It is hard on whoever's body it is in; hard on the loved ones of whoever's body it is in; hard on so many people around whoever's body it is in. Cancer IS hard and shouldn't be made to look easy. I don't want to wear a pink anything to show the world I have breast cancer. I wish there was no pink anything for anyone to wear so that would mean no one had breast cancer. Now don't get me wrong, there are "pretty" things that do come out of cancer: You can find yourself. Your real self that you never knew was in there, your strong self that God fills with life day after day. You can help people find compassion for others. You can help people realize EVERYONE is going through something no matter how pretty perfect they look on the outside. You meet this whole new subgroup of people that truly understand your pain. You learn to say yes and no to what your heart is really telling you to do. It is scary to do, even when you are sick. What if someone gets mad at you? You learn if they get mad at you, their love for themselves is greater than their love for others and it is okay to let that person go. You learn life is FULL of the unknown and how to truly be thankful for each day. Even if it is a feel bad day, a day you lay on the couch all day or a day you are able to do everything you want to do. You learn to thank God for every second of everyday because you truly don't know what will happen next. You learn not to try to plan life out because again you don't know what will happen next. YOUR plan really means nothing in the grand scheme of things.

What is breast cancer to me - part 2 – June 14, 2013

I don't get the whole "I will kick this cancer's ass mentality" so many of us have. Don't get me wrong here, I think we all need to go into this as if it were a WAR...BUT if you only have fight on your heart all the time, you will miss a lot, a lot that needs to be learned from this fight. I feel like with this mentality running all over the place especially with young women. We forget to learn to be easy on ourselves. We look at getting chemo, radiation, surgeries, etc. as more of a *to-do list*. These are NOT normal things to add to a to-do list. It seems we just add this *stuff* to our lists, but we don't stop, think and feel what is happening? I didn't until after it was over the first time. My first time through chemo, I pushed through trying to keep up the image I was fine. I was in control and it was no big deal to get eight rounds of chemo in 16 weeks; followed by a lumpectomy and biopsy right after that. Oh yeah, add a cruise on to that list. It was good, but it was hard. My body was tired and depression started to set in, but why depression now? I was CLEAN?!?!

Then came the 37 treatments of radiation. Some people say radiation is a breeze, but it sure wasn't for me. It completely zapped my energy, and I felt guilty for this because it was "supposed" to be easy. All through this whole process, I kept that thought, "but I will kick this cancer's ass." I felt if I wasn't in constant fight mode, I wasn't doing what needed to be done. But what I didn't realize was, one can't survivor in fight mode ALL the time. Once the exterior of fight/hard edge/I am bad ass mode started to crack, I realized fight mode wasn't/isn't for me all the time. When you are going through treatment just know you don't have to be superwomen. You don't have to keep up your "old life" and just add treatment to your to-do list. It isn't just a to-do. It is a life changing point and you should embrace it as such.

What is breast cancer to me - part 3 – June 18, 2013

I have noticed a trend when someone is newly diagnosed with whatever life changing disease, as soon as we tell people we have been diagnosed with the big C word, most of our family, friends and acquaintances in our lives rally around us telling us we can do this. We can beat this. We've got this in the bag, etc. All of which I believe, all of which I think is awesome to vocalize this support to one and other. But, my question is, why do we wait to tell each other these wonderful words of encouragement, faith in one another, uplifting words? Why do we wait until a diagnosis like this to tell each other what strong, inspirational, awesome people we think each other is? And this isn't just about breast cancer. Why don't we tell each other these things on an on-going basis? Why is it scary to tell someone who we think is awesome that we think they are awesome, that we think they are so strong and can overcome whatever, that they did an amazing job at something, that they are a Godly person through and through, that one time they told you something that really changed you. Why don't we tell people in our lives these things? Why do we wait for a tragedy to hit someone we know before we say these things?

Just to be clear, I do this too! I think we wait because it is scary. We think, oh shit, what if they don't tell us the same thing back. BUT the thing is, when we tell people these things, we shouldn't expect the person we are telling these things to say it back. We should tell people these things because we believe them in our hearts and we want to share this love with the other person, plain and simple. Back to breast cancer, when I was diagnosed both times people came out of the woodwork telling me what a strong person I have always been, if anyone had this it was me, I had a smile that lit up a room, I was such a great God loving person, SO many heartwarming things. I had this cancer thing in the bag. And I have noticed this with so many newly diagnosed people they all hear these wonderful words of encouragement too. Which is great. But my question is, why don't we all tell each other these things ALL the time? Not just when we get horrible news? Why don't we tell each other how awesome we think each other are all the time?

I admit it; it did take cancer for me to get this. To get that we should encourage, love, forgive all of it, all the time. And not wait until we are scared and don't know what is coming next. Do it now. So, what I propose is that when you get the feeling to tell someone that they are awesome, that you believe in someone for something, that you see an awesome trait someone has, that you see someone do something so sweet for someone else, that you think someone is a great parent, tell them. Tell them all those little things that run through your head. Those little things you think of them, those things that you think make them be such an awesome person...tell them!! Don't wait until a tragedy strikes, tell them these things ALL the time...it is an amazing thing for both you and them!!

"The most important thing in life is to learn how to give out love, and to let it come in." – Morrie Schwartz

Radiation…it is catching up with me – June 20, 2013

I am tired.

I am not able to sleep a whole night.

I have a small lingering headache most of the time which makes me blah.

BUT, after seeing the radiation doctor on Tuesday, I feel great about where I am at. He said he is very happy with how great I look and for my next appointment with him I don't even have to go in, I can just call in and let him know all is well. Let me set the record straight though, I have earned this right with these doctors because they totally trust me from the past. They know I will tell them when something is wrong. My hair is starting to hurt, so I know it will start falling out soon. I can't decide if I want to shave it all vs. having a big ole bald spot?? I still have constant constipation issues no matter how well I eat, or how many chia seeds I put in my smoothies. I still need to take laxatives, but oh well! I have what they call "moon face" from the steroids. Thank goodness they told me I could stop taking them on Tuesday. BUT compared to my first time radiation, this is 100% better and I will take what I have now versus what I had then any day.

"If you tell the truth you don't have to remember anything." – Mark Twain

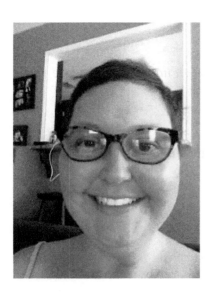

Can I get off this merry go-round now?? – June 23, 2013

I feel like I am on a merry go-round...all the time, up and down, round and round, up and down, round and round...forever going on...I just want off for a little bit...but then I wonder, what would happen if I did get off? Aren't we all on a merry go-round, isn't that life??

I had to go back to the ER on Friday because my whole right side went numb and this time I had a twitch added to it, a twitch in my right upper leg that would not stop, probably lasted three hours total and finally stopped when they gave me an IV steroid and muscle relaxer. When I first called my radiation doctor to see what they wanted me to do, he said ER because he was afraid it might be a stroke. But I was 99% sure it wasn't and it was just brain swelling again, but I wasn't going to be 100% until I had a CT scan. The ER was a total cluster -the admin lady...well, let's just say IF I were having a stroke, well, I am not sure how that would have turned out.

After WAY TOO long in my opinion, she got me checked in. I GUESS she could tell by my speech and ability to smile I wasn't having a stroke...but it still took a LONG time. Got back, talked to the same ER doctor who had to tell me the first time that it was a tumor (yes he remembered me), got blood drawn, IV hooked up, then a trauma case came in, so I had to wait another 30 minutes or so until my other RN got there and then she came in and gave me my medication. I finally stopped shaking and calmed down due to medication. Got my CT scan, all was clear!! So this was all caused from the swelling, so I am back on steroids...lovely!

I am completely worn down. I think the radiation is taking full effect now, hence the swelling again. I have slept on and off most of the day Saturday and today and am still tired. I am tired of being tired, but oh well; it is what it is at this point. I kind of sort of had

Eric shave my head this morning. My hair is really falling out and it hurts and it is just easier with it so short. So be it. We leave this week to go up to Eric's family lake house in MI and I am so looking forward to that! Here is to keepin' on keepin' on

The Knock... - June 30, 2013

Knowing the sound

of the Knock

that Precious knock

Knowing all I needed to do

was open the door

The door that seemed

to have been bolted shut

for way too long

The door...

I admit I have cracked it open

Just a sliver...

a small sliver

from time to time

Always

too afraid

to fling it open wide open

Not knowing what was on the other side

But

the Knock continued

day and night —

always

Some days

it would drive me crazy

I would try anything

to make it stop

Other days

I would entertain

the idea

of possibly

maybe

opening

The door

One day...

My heart won

the battle of the day

I let my heart

have its way

I let my heart

open the door

I was tired

Tired of fighting...

Fighting to keep

the door closed

To keep

my heart in the dark

To keep

me where I was...

A light so bright

Joy so intense

Peace so calming

Love so burning

was on the other side

God smiled at me

and said,

"I've been waiting...

for you"

To the care givers – July 3, 2013

I would like to take this chance to say thank you to all the care givers out there. So many people tell me and others going through a disease what an inspiration we are to them, but I think a lot of people forget a HUGE part of this equation is the care givers.

The ones who are with us through it all: the news, the plans, the process of it all, every part of the journey.

They hold our hands when we get bad news all while holding themselves together.

They hold our hands while getting treatments, tests, IV pokes and so much more.

They hold the weight of their own world, our world, our children's world, all on their shoulders, all the time.

They keep their live going all while balancing this new life thrown at them also.

They are the gatekeeper between the patient and outside world. To protect us from others, others who don't intentionally harm us with their words or actions, but we need a gatekeeper.

I realize way too many patients aren't as blessed as I am. I not only have my wonderful husband who I can't imagine going through this journey without, but he can't imagine letting me go through any of this on my own. I have my family and friends also, who circle around me and cover me with love whenever they can. I believe we all need to be givers daily. Even if we aren't care givers in a traditional sense we need to all be givers in any sense to those in the world daily. When you see someone who needs a hand, lend it. So what if it is a homeless person and they are asking for a $1 and you don't know what they will spend it on. If you can help him/her at that point in time, do it!

When you see someone who needs love, give it, even if it is just with a smile. When you see a friend is in need, do all you can to help.

When you see an empty space in the world that needs to be filled, fill it with love and kindness. I know it sounds like a big task, but it doesn't have to be. Start small. Something is better is nothing in any sense.

Good bye my friend – July 10, 2013

"I can't change the direction of the wind, but I can adjust my sails to reach my destination." – Jimmy Dean.

I hate cancer....really, I hate it.

One of the girls who I have been on this whole Cancerland adventure with this whole time passed away last night from fucking cancer.

I can say so much and so little right now about it all.

As in most large groups of people, there was a smaller group. Us three, all around 35, stage IV breast cancer, fun loving girls trying to live our lives without cancer getting too much in the way.

We did it.

We all did it for two and a half years...until now...we aren't all doing it anymore.

It all happened so fast.

Casey was beautiful and had a smile that would light up a room.

We would talk about everything from making totally inappropriate comments to each other about cancer and laugh.

How we were afraid of dying, how we didn't understand why cancer attacked our bodies, our poo issues, the stress we feel about trying to balance life in Cancerland while keeping one foot in the real world, how easy it would be to let Cancerland swallow us up.

I never asked her if she wanted kids. It seemed unkind. I knew what the answer was at this point in time.

I never asked her what her dreams were before this cancer bullshit. I don't know why. I guess I knew her unspoken dream, to have her cancer be gone.

She did get the Jeep she always wanted but sure didn't get enough time to enjoy *the hell out of it* like she wanted.

We talked about God and how hard it is to keep faith through all of this, through so much.

I am all out of words. My hearts hurts...it hurts for so much...so much.

Today is going to be a hard day. Another funeral of someone who was much too young. It is so hard because I KNOW what great friends we could have been if we were to meet at a different point in our lives. We were great friends for the little time we knew each other, but I know there was more to our friendship.

Nothing makes sense to me right now. I feel like cancer is the Cheshire Cat in my own personal Cancerland, it shows up when it wants to, it disappears now and then.

From Alice In Wonderland:

"Would you tell me, please, which way I ought to go from here?" "That depends a good deal on where you want to get to," said the Cat. "I don't much care where –" said Alice. "Then it doesn't matter which way you go," said the Cat. "– so long as I get somewhere," Alice added as an explanation. "Oh, you're sure to do that," said the Cat, "if you only walk long enough."

The cat is an enigma, perhaps symbolizing the mystery of Wonderland itself, of how nonsense has a way of making sense. The Cheshire cat to me is the one character of Wonderland who does make a little bit of sense to me. He knows he's mad. I guess kind of like we all know we are going to die at some point, but never thought we would think about it like this. It consumes you. The cat comes and he goes, he is and he isn't, he's there then he's not....When the queen tries to behead the cat, he disappears, but his head remains and he asks, "Can something that does not have a body be beheaded?" So yes, cancer itself is the cat.

Does it even have a body?

MRI and brain oncologist – July 12, 2013

MRI was clear and all looks great! I was even able to follow up with my radiation doctor on the phone being as it all looked so good. NOW that is what I like! We went to see Groves yesterday. He sent in some of my original breast tumor and some of my brain tumor marker analysis. Let me just tell you science is CRAZY and anyone who thinks, oh, just eat better and it will cure your cancer is just plain WRONG! Here is how I understood it, Eric might read it and leave a whole list of different things to add! So, my original breast cancer started with mutation in 3 areas, let's call them A, B and C. My breast cancer in my brain has 5 mutations, we'll call them A, B, D, E and F So somewhere along the way, my body go rid of C but the cancer adapted to that and grew D, E and F. The good news is, there are drugs that cross the blood brain barrier that work on some of these...we can't work on all of them at once. BUT we have choices.

As of now we have two choices. I am reading about the possible side effects and will go from there. One choice we will leave in our bag of tricks just in case we need it further down the line, it is a skin cancer chemo. All in all, we left Dr. G's office feeling great. He did tell me I was a very "neat" case. I guess if you are into that stuff I do seem neat?!?! He and Eric had as great time at the white board drawing cell path ways. Once we told him Eric was an EE, he was like, this is just like that. One circuit closes and another opens. I still don't know what that means!? But I have my PET scan today and am really anxious for those results. I haven't been on anything for two months and to say I am not at all nervous would be a total lie.

Nervous... - July 17, 2013

I go see Dr. H today to find out what my next path will be. I go back and forth within myself. *Am I ready to be back on a chemo?* In a way yes because I feel like I am more protected, especially with my brain. In a way, HELL NO I am not ready for the unknown. The fatigue, poo issues, appetite, nausea, all these are "maybe" side effects and those I won't know until I have already jumped in. On a plus side, my face is starting de-swell from the 'roids!

New chemo – July 18, 2013

I must say, it was odd to leave Dr. H's office with a bag full of chemo pills, odd as in crazy. Eric and I joked when we went to lunch that we shouldn't leave the chemo in the car, after the pharmacist telling Eric we are SO lucky to have the insurance we have being as two weeks of this little beauty can be a pretty penny. I am now on Xeloda. I will take four pills in the morning and four at night; Two weeks on and a week off. The major side effect of this chemo seems to be dry, pealing and cracked hands and feet. They say it will be like farmers dry/cracked hands. I am going to get some gloves and footy boots to put thick cream on in the morning and night to help combat this. There are the possible other side effects: vomiting, diarrhea, nausea, sores in mouth BUT most of those are "not common." I will let y'all know how it goes! I am going to paint today a commission for a 1st birthday and I am SO excited to be able to lose myself in paint!

The truth... – July 22, 2013

Ian asked me if there was any such thing as a real happy place. I told him of course. In your heart and mind you can always be in your happy place.

People tell me all the time that we handle "all this" so well that they don't think they could handle it like Eric and I do. I tell everyone the same thing, yes you could, there is nothing special about me. I just allow my heart to shine through more than some others. As humans I think our first response to anything is to put a wall up, shelter our hearts, and put on any kind of armor we can find to protect ourselves. From what, well whatever is attacking us! I just want to remind everyone that you too, YES YOU TOO have it in you to fight whatever battle it is that you are fighting. Some days, you might have to take a day off; some days, you have to give yourself time to morn whatever it is you are going through; but when that voice says you can't do anymore or you aren't strong enough that is when you HAVE to listen to your heart.

Our heart's voice it is a tiny voice compared to the loud yelling of the other voice saying you can't. But you can. Even if you can only take a twelfth of a step forward for however many days, you must keep stepping forward. I was complaining to Eric yesterday about me not being able to walk long distances because it has been almost a year since surgery. He laughed and said NO, it has been almost a year since surgery ONE and you reset that for surgery TWO and reset again for surgery THREE. So really you are at two months post-surgery. I let that loud voice speak instead of my heart. It always makes me laugh when I look back on things like this and I am amazed at how hard on myself I am. Which I know we all are that hard on ourselves. But the thing is, would we ever expect others to do this crazy shit we ask out of ourselves? NO. Remember that the next time that loud voice starts in on you, stop and listen to your heart for the truth.

I am tired... – July 27, 2013

I am tired of this weird rash on the bottom of my legs that itches like crazy unless I take Benadryl, which then makes me pass out. I could take a steroid, but I would rather itch being as I am JUST NOW starting to lose some of the water weight. Dr. H told me to hold my chemo for the weekend. But now I am a little worried about not being on my chemo this weekend. I still don't have energy all day long. I can go a few hours, but then I crash. It sucks to have this "want to do" list, but never getting it a quarter of the way done. My patience is gone at 6:00pm and it sucks because I haven't been with Ian or Eric most of the day, but I am just so tired in the evening my patience just vanishes. I have really been working on not being grumping towards them. I think I might need to start PT again. My walking with this wonky limp is making my knee hurt. I am tired of not having feeling in my whole left leg. I am tired of having to have Eric do everything physical. I SO want to help him move our stuff to the new house, and him not have all this weight on his shoulders, for me to be his other half. I feel more like a growth that he has to lug around versus a helping partner. Blah, I am just blah. Luckily we have a birthday party to go to today and all my friends will be there too. Really, I think we throw our kids these birthday parties for us mommies to get together. Whatever, the kids are happy! OH, and us too!!

Opening Up – August 5, 2013

I need to start practicing opening up more. I do good sometimes at letting it all hang out, then just like a switch being turned off, my heart closes up and decides I am done being that open. Being open is a scary place. People can attack so easily because you are letting it all hang out, which I think is a beautiful thing. I have spent so much time building this façade that all is great with me all the time, when in reality it isn't, but I am now realizing that it isn't with anyone. SO, here is me starting to really open up. If you wish to join me, please do so.

What is praying to you? Praying to me is just talking to God like I do a friend. Sometime I ask Him for help, sometimes I just unload on Him. Sometime I ask what He needs from me just like I do a friend.

How often do you pray? I go through cycles. I used to only pray when shit hit the fan, but only AFTER I tried to solve it myself. Then I go through phases where I pray all the time about everything. Then somehow I forget to do that, so I do back to the other way.

I now put a bright sticky note in random places to remind me to pray through the day, I love it like this.

Do you have a prayer time and place? I tried this but it didn't work. I tried to do it first thing in the morning, but sometimes I would forget. I tried to do it right before bed, but sometimes I fell asleep before I got it all out. So now, I do it whenever/wherever I feel the need to talk to Him.

Do you tend to only pray when shit hits the fan? Like I said before I used to be like this. Of course when I was diagnosed the first time, I was on my knees all the time. Then I got better, and the urge to talk went away. Don't get me wrong, I would pray on and off, but nothing consistent. Then another switch flipped, now my heart tells me I need more day to day contact, so I pray throughout the day. If I see a wreck, I pray for the people involved and people there to help. If I see a homeless person, I pray for them. At red lights, I pray for the people around me. When someone pops into my head, I pray for them. I like this way much better!

Dear Ian – August 14, 2013

Yes, I will say this every year, but I can NOT believe you are 6. We have had a wild year around here. We went to California to visit BeBe and Aunt Tam. We went to Disney Land, Lego Land and Hollywood. I had three brain surgeries, big BB lived with us for about 5 months and we moved to a new house. And through all of this, you were such a trooper. You amaze me daily with your love, kindness and ability to make us laugh. You have had this attitude lately that I am working on, showing you have a happy heart. Some days are better than others, but that is one of my jobs as your mommy to show you how to respect and be kind to others even if you don't feel like it. Other than the 'tude, you are so sweet. You started karate this summer at camp, and went in it not knowing anyone, but you have made lots of friends, which makes me so happy for you. You are easy going and love to make others laugh. You excel in math and we have math wars with each other which is always fun. It is so much fun to watch you grow and see you are growing into.

I love you,

Mommy

Breaking – August 16, 2013

I feel like I am breaking, breaking from lack of control. I am not one who really gives a shit if someone does something how I think it should be done, but our home life has been so crazy these past few weeks. I think it is all catching up to me. We have moved to our new house, but both houses are a wreck. We are having a garage sale tomorrow and anything that doesn't go, will go straight to Goodwill. I am DONE with all this extra shit. We are waiting for our new countertop, so the kitchen is a complete mess. I have been eating like crap and feel it because I can't cook. My painting space is in boxes and I want to cry. I did cry. Many times that past few days from lack of control, from feeling so tired ALL the time, from it all. I cried.

Whole Heart – August 21, 2013

It is easy –

to say "I believe"

to say "I love"

but with my whole heart?

my whole soul?

Isn't that mine

to keep

all for me?

To give it away -

For free

For love?

Have I ever loved like that...

with my whole heart?

I know the feeling of pure love:

Holding a sleeping child.

Holding a loved one's hand

A tight hug from a friend

a warm Wash of

Comfort

Love

Peace

settles into your heart.

Into the cracks you didn't know where there

But in that moment

you know

Pure love

God's love

What if

we remember

that Love

that Feeling

And in return

love God

with that Love?

love each other

with that Love?

First day of kindergarten - August 25, 2013

Oh my sweet little Ian. I can't really say little anymore because you are taller than any 6 year old I know, but you will always be my little man no matter how big or old you are. You start kindergarten tomorrow and I must say I am more nervous than you are, or you are hiding it really well. As far as I know, you don't know anyone in your class because I decided to go against the grain and not put you in the bi-lingual class with all your friends. You might not be thanking me for this for a few weeks, but I truly believe this is the best for you to just do it, jump in with both feet and not hold back. I know you are great at making new friends. You went to karate camp all summer where you didn't know one person at the beginning and ended up with lots friends at the end.

My sweet boy, I pray for you to be kind and compassionate to all, no matter what. I know there will be some not so great times ahead and I pray that you listen to your heart and let it guide you and not to peer-pressure. Being liked by everyone, especially the ones who are mean to others is no way to want to go through life. I pray that your light shines through to all who cross your path. I pray for you to have strength and courage in all you do. Most of all I pray for love, for you, for your friends, teachers and all others who will get to be with you all day. I pray that you are all surrounded by and show love to all. My sweet boy, I love you

Happy Anniversary?!?! - August 30, 2013

I can't say I am one who remembers or even really talk about any of my "cancerversaries" (notice this is plural...as in too many to remember). But today is one I couldn't let slip by without talking about. One year ago today, right about this time, I was being told I had a large mass in my brain, large as in more than 5 cm.

That yes, my cancer had once again decided to try to move to a residence in my body.

That yes I would need brain surgery.

That yes the family was coming to Austin to be here with us.

That yes once again, our sweet family was going to be rocked in ways we never knew were possible.

In one short year, I have had three brain surgeries, two brain radiations, countless doses of chemo, changed chemo drugs, been on steroids too many times and I am sure there is stuff I am forgetting. (You know because of the three brain surgeries and all.) This year tore layers off of me I didn't know were there to be torn.

There were days I was pretty sure I would never really be cancer free.

There were days I didn't want to try anymore. I didn't want to try to live this new life that had been thrown at me with no one asking me if I was ok with it. I was ready to throw in towel one way or another.

This past year has hands down been the hardest year of my life. But I don't want to live my life around my cancer calendar. We have also traveled, moved into a new house, watched Ian graduate Pre-K, walked him to and from kinder daily, been with friends and family and just enjoy life. Some days I get all worked up about some small something. I am not eating enough veggies, the kitchen is still a mess from this morning (right now actually), I can only do one "major" activity a day without being beat down tired, I am looking into the guest room that is still piled high with moving boxes, but then I snap out of it and remember who cares at least I don't have another brain tumor!

40 is the new 30...not in Cancerland – September 15, 2013

In my world, 35 is the new 50, with menopause and all. I had wondered about this for a while. If I was in menopause or close to it? A simple blood test later said yes, yes I am on the tail end side of pre-memo pause. Nice. And now I can once and for all say I am truly sorry for being a snappy bitch lately, my hormones are making me do it. And yes, when I started crying the other day for NO reason, again the hormones. No sleeping through the night for me, check. Irritability, BIG CHECK. Hot Flashes, had those a few months ago but I chalked it up to radiation after effects, it could have been a double whammy? Crashing fatigue, anxiety, mental confusion, itchy skin, check, check, check and check. Now these I still chalk up to recent surgery and new chemo, but I could be wrong?? What if once I do go through full menopause I am a whole new person, with this new memory and energy? Well you are right, menopause isn't going to give me back that part of my life. I am curious to see how this all plays out.

Pink, pink, pink – everywhere is pink. – September 19, 2013

It might make you think everything is Pretty in Pink. I wish it was... truly, I do.

It isn't tough.

I am not one to really rock the boat most of the time that is, but if you push me enough I will break. And this is me breaking.

I am sick of pink.

This post is going to be a bit of a soapbox rant with a purpose! I don't want to wear pink to announce to the world that I have breast cancer...I want to wear pink because it is one of my favorite colors.

I don't want a pink can opener or some other gadget to help me show my support of breast cancer.

What does that mean anyway? How exactly are you showing support with all these pink items??

I am sick of companies selling stuff in pink and giving off the impression that a large percent of the money goes to cancer patients or research.

The kicker is, we don't even know what part of breast cancer that tiny percent goes to. It could go to making more products to "support" breast cancer? I am just speculating here SO don't get offended by this. I think we are ALL aware of breast cancer. I mean, if the stats don't lie then 1 in 8 women will have it. For it not to affect everyone on some level is pretty much impossible.

Another question - where does that money go? Does it go to the little people who need help during their battle?? When I say little people, I mean the ones who make just enough not to qualify for government help but get diagnosed with cancer? What happens to them and all this money raised?

From what I hear, they (the "little people") are made to jump through hoops to get only a little bit of help. Let me tell you, as a stage IV breast cancer "thriver," doing paperwork with chemo brain is not only mentally exhausting, it is next to impossible. So now, you have someone who is stressed from the cancer diagnosis, working, getting chemo treatment, taking care of a family, and in order to get a little help with the bills, is expected to fill out lengthy forms! And yes, I get it. I realize we can't just hand out cash to everyone, BUT every once in a while there is a story that touches you and you KNOW you have to help in some way. That is why I am asking you to *think before you pink* this year. If you are going to spend money to help the cause, I am asking you to help this young woman instead of buying "pink stuff," since we aren't really sure where the proceeds it goes to.

The girl who cried wolf... - October 1, 2013

Or maybe something else instead... I guess having a small seizure is still a good reason to rush off to the ER and MUCH better than getting told my cancer is back in the brain.

Small update from yesterday: the right side of my face and head started going numb and then my right leg started twitching uncontrollably. I called Eric; Dr. H wanted an MRI stat...went to the ER; no cancer!!! I had a small seizure so I will follow up with Dr. Cutie next week.

I feel completely beat down tired today, but the show must go on. I have a TV interview this afternoon about my thoughts on the cure. Ian has parkour; and that is it for today. I still need to practice my speech more for Thursday night, but I will do that soon too. I feel like whatever is going on has been one of the reasons I have been SO FLIPPING beat down tired. I have no energy to do anything more than be with Ian and Eric. I have to miss too many events lately and it sucks, but when it comes down to it, I would rather have this energy for Ian. SO for now, onward and upward!

Speech – October 2013

I was asked to speak at the "Be Brave, Fight like a girl" fundraiser event to benefit Heal in Comfort.

It was great to be there – up on stage telling my story, knowing I was touching hearts and helping raise money for a great cause.

Of course, I totally crashed today...oh well.

Playing Poker with breast cancer – October 15, 2013

October is a hard month for me. Actually all months are hard months for me. As I see others celebrate their victory over cancer, it is all too easy for my mind to slip to that dark place and wonder what did they do that I didn't do, should I have prayed more, should I have never eaten laffy-taffy, was it caused because I smoked, did Pantex have something to do with it?

All these questions run through my mind when I see others post about fighting breast cancer and winning. Then I wonder if maybe I just didn't fight hard enough the first time. But that is the word that bothers me about this all, fight. I feel like it implies that those who are done with cancer fought and won versus those or aren't ever done didn't fight quite hard enough.

After much back and forth with myself, I have settled on this: Cancer is like playing Texas Hold 'em, stay with me here. Let's say you have 4 players at the table. The cards are dealt. You first look at the cards and moan and groan and think there is nothing to be made from this hand and the whole way through the hand it is hard to watch and stay in, but there is something in you telling you to hang in and bet big on the last card. You do and you end up with a full boat. You are elated with success! You had to hang in and sweat it out, but the outcome is *winner, winner chicken dinner*. You gather your winnings and head home. But for me and too many other stage IV-ers, we were forced back in the game. A game we never wanted to play again. Some of us won that first hand too only to be made to play again. You did not choose to be put back into the game and you sure as hell didn't get back in it by not eating the right thing, standing on our hands 10 minutes a day, or some other crazy notion someone always wants to tell you about. If you would have done this or that you wouldn't be where you are now. To me, being stage IV is just like repeatedly getting dealt bad hands. Nothing we stage IV-ers did to deserve these bad hands, nothing you did to deserve your winning hand. It is luck of the draw and is what it is.

Is this my new life?? – October 23, 2013

The flash back

the heart stop

the deflated feeling

the swirls in your head

in your heart every time...

every single time someone you care about someone you might not know

but are connected to

connected to by more than this disease just when one heart heals

another heart breaks

those shards pierce us all

it feels like we will never have a whole heart again

Killer headaches equals nothing good – December 6, 2013

I had to get an MRI Tuesday because I have been having horrible headaches that are making me feel sick to my stomach. I found out yesterday there is something there, but they think it is just dead tissue. All I know at this point is Groves is looking at it all and I will get an appointment with him hopefully Monday to figure out next steps. Until then I started back on the 'roids yesterday, oh boy! To try to make the swelling go down and make these damn headaches go away. I will let you know what happens next.

Doctor report - December 17, 2013

This isn't as much information as I had hoped and prayed for going into the meeting yesterday but, it is what it is. He bumped my steroids in hopes of getting the swelling down saying that it was concerning that I had been on steroids for a week and I still have these headaches Still no one knows if it's necrosis or a tumor as nobody will be able to tell without surgery.

I do have a PET scan scheduled for Monday. Until then I am just taking it easy and treating it like a massive migraine. I wish there was more, I wish I had a plan...I don't.

More than anything I want my head not to hurt.

The plan as I understand it: We will up the steroids this week if that doesn't bring down the swelling, we will try Avastin (different chemo) which could possibly get rid of some of the necrotic issue. And if that doesn't work, then we go into surgery and go from there. So there's a lot of if's, and's, or but's to rule out stuff. Best case scenario, it is only dead swelling tissues (yes I will take it). Worst case scenario, surgery. We have lots more to try before it comes to that.

I am tired of being tired, of hurting and not knowing...but it is what it is.

Update on Renee – December 31, 2013

Hi everyone, this is Eric writing for Renee. Renee has been having a lot of ups and downs lately, but the constant has been a very heavy fatigue and headaches. She can't really focus very long, and staring at a computer screen to type really hurts her head. She sends her regrets on not being able to talk, write or be around for everyone, but appreciates all the well wishes, thoughts and prayers. The past week or two we have been very worried that there was more tumor growth due to all the issues she was having. But then she had a MRI on Friday Dec 27th, and then we met with the Neuro-Oncologist on Monday the 30th. Prayers were answered, and the latest MRI shows that the swelling is coming down, and there's nothing that indicates an active tumor. The most likely thing is necrosis from the surgeries and the multiple radiation treatments to the same area. It seems strange to us that it would show up as symptoms so long after the actual treatments, but we will take necrosis over tumor any day. That being said, it still doesn't explain why Renee is feeling so bad still, or how to give her any relief. The only thing that seems to help her for now is lots of rest while her body heals.

The current plan is that since the swelling seems to be going down, she's on a taper to get off the steroids, which hopefully will help with some of the fatigue. Renee had a PET scan planned for before Christmas, but the machine broke a half hour before she was scheduled. So, now she has a PET scan over her whole body on Thursday to make sure she's still clean everywhere else, and then we'll meet with her regular Oncologist on Friday. Assuming that her PET scan is clear and that she's not improved from being off the steroids, there's still the possibility of being on Avastin to help with the inflammation in her brain. It would be an IV drip for her, but no side effects that would make her feel worse than she does. In the meantime, she's still on her oral chemo, as well as pain and nausea meds to keep everything in check. Her spirits are up and down, but with the MRI news we're all a lot more hopeful about turning a corner soon. More than anything, she's just tired of feeling tired and hurting, and ready to get back to feeling like herself. We'll update things here as we get more information, and thank you everyone again for the thoughts and prayers. We wish everyone a happy new year and may 2014 find you and yours with an abundance of Joy and Love throughout the year.

2014

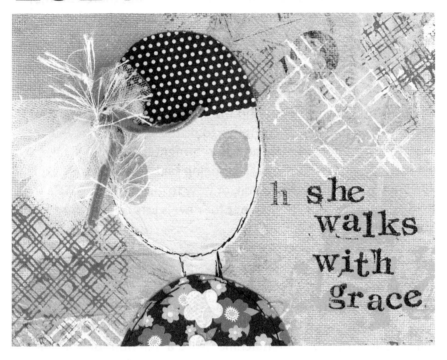

h s he
walks
with
grace

PET! – January 4, 2014

Hi all, it's Eric writing for Renee again, wanting to update everyone on how she's doing. She started off the New Year with a PET scan on Thursday the 2nd, and a follow up with Dr. H yesterday. Even though we were really worried about her bones & lungs because of some pains and issues, the PET was clear! That was the best possible outcome, and we had to hear it a few times to believe it, and are thanking God so much for what seems like a true miracle. As expected, they weren't able to get a lot of information about her head from the PET, just from the way the PET actually works. But that wasn't a big deal, and we'll just take the good results from the previous MRIs. Her symptoms are unfortunately still there, and she's feeling very run down and still has some pain in her body and her head. But, we're still very stoked to know the scans are looking good, and are looking forward to getting everything figured out and her feeling better.

Based on the scans, the working assumption is that her symptoms are caused by necrosis in her brain from her surgeries and radiation, as well as some symptoms from the side effects of her steroids. So, she's getting off the steroids, which will hopefully help with the energy levels & some of the body pains. Then she'll also be starting a new treatment of Avastin next Friday, which should help with the head pain and help her deal with the necrosis. She'll also stay on her current chemo. All in all, it's a great start to the New Year, and we're looking forward to having her feel better. We thank everyone for all the help, thoughts and prayers as we get things back on track.

Spinal tap and more – January 23, 2014

I had my first and hopefully last ever spinal tap on Monday. Now I "thought" this was going to be easy breezy, a small poke and fluid draw…I thought WRONG. The PA did it, so she went lower because that is a less risky area and come to find out a harder area to get. The numbing poke didn't hurt too much. So I was supposed to be all numbed …I wasn't. She had to dig around to hit the fluid, in the process a few nerves were hit and I am pretty sure that was the worst pain ever and that is what sent me over the edge. I don't know how many digs into my spine later before she got me some good drugs? We let those kick in, got Groves in there to do the tap and BAM, he got it on the first stick. He went up higher on my spine which is risky but I didn't feel it due to the new pain meds kicking in. So after all that, I could barely walk out due to the meds and shots. I went home and passed out. Then later in the week I found out it was all worth it, ALL IS GREAT!! No cancer cells lurking around in my spinal fluid.

I have a follow up MRI next Thursday but I am starting to feel better. My head just hurts when I am tired, but it hurts less than it did!!

I am going to start practicing driving the parking lot this weekend. I am also hoping that I don't get car sick and the two leg driving comes back easily! So all in all, things are going well. Thanks for all the prayers and love.

Where do I go from here?? – February 25, 2014

A few years ago, it would have seemed to me that I would be ecstatic to be where I am now, alive and well, it would seem to me that I should be able to go from doom and gloom to delight and praise at the flip of a switch. Some secret internal switch that I should be able to switch back and forth with ease, or at least switch back and forth a few days after good news.

I am not sure my switch works anymore.

I am pretty sure my switch has become numb to these emotions.

I seem to stay either in the middle of the road of emotions leaning more to I don't care.

It isn't that I don't care how I am feeling because believe me I do, but it is becoming increasingly harder to get too vested and comfy/cozy at any certain point of how I feel because once I seem to be comfortable at any one point (either good or bad) the rug is yanked out from under me once again and I tumble to the ground, along with all the other things that are leaned up against me.

It is getting harder and harder to get back up, dust myself off and take a step forward. It is great when I feel good, but I seem to have put a fence around me that I can't climb over to the other side where feeling great is...even to where feeling good is. I can see the fence and over the fence, but I can't touch it much less grab ahold of it and climb it to the other side.

I feel like my true peace of mind is on that other side. That true piece of heart and mind I long to have again, true peace of heart and mind that I used to have; true peace of heart and mind that used to shine though me even when all I could see was miles and miles of shit ahead of me. I used to trust it would all truly go back to "normal." I still trust it will, but I am learning it never goes back as quick as I pray for it to or to exactly where it was before. My "normal" changes every day, I never know what I am going to wake up and feel like, I never know if I am going to have another seizure (or whatever you want to call them) that seems to throw my whole world out of control for weeks to months on end. The harder I try to hang on to control the faster I seem to spin...spin down. I feel like with all this spinning, so many pieces of me are scattered all over the place. I used to be able to see where the pieces landed sweep them all back up in a pile and somewhat put them, put me back together. But now, I seem to have lost sight of so many of the pieces. I don't even know where to begin looking to start the sweeping up process yet again. I am not sure where the road leads from here.

3 years – March 12, 2014

It will be 3 years ago on Friday that I got the call I never wanted to get. The call I honestly never thought was possible to get again. Yes, I was naïve back then, I lived in my peaceful ignorance is bliss bubble. Hey, I was happy there! I didn't take the time to educate myself on what could happen, because in my mind if I knew what could happen then that fear would consume me, like it sometimes does now because let's be honest I am all too familiar with what can happen. It seems to happen to me all the time. I can easily say never in a million years could I have imaged this scenario of a shit show as my life. I don't really want to recap what has happened in the past 3 years, it is what it is.

I will one of these days.

It has been harder than hard at some points, sometimes I honestly didn't know how I would continue on living the life I have been handed, I probably have cried enough tears to fill a swimming pool (or maybe not that many), I have had to relearn to walk with one numb leg, type, write, paint and so much more not once but twice, I keep having to learn how to live my new life that is me for now.

I try hard not to freak out and crumble every time I have a headache or a new pain in my body that isn't easily explained away.

I try hard not to get mad at God when things start going really bad.

I try to forgive myself for not being the mom, wife, daughter, sister, friend that I want to be, but to be completely honest I am not really sure I ever was as "great" as I remember myself being. Who knows?

I try hard to go easy on myself for all the weight I have gained from steroids.

I try hard not to compare my story to other's stories, and have finally accepted all of our stories are completely different and that is ok, even good. What would we talk about if all of our stories were the same?

So here I am, three years later. Still trying to make sense of it all, continuing to dig through the rubble and once again rebuilding myself. Some say that is a miracle in itself being as a lot of others don't survive three years past their breast cancer metastasizing. I say it is God's plan, even though I am mad at Him half the time, I do realize there is a Plan.

Wide open – March 24, 2014

I often toe the line while writing for my blog. I give y'all a glimpse into my world, but I don't ever fully open the door for the outside world to see in to me. But, I think I have to. I think I have to 100% swing the door wide open, if I am truly hoping for others to understand where I and so many others actually do stand. To help you understand how it feels to be in my shoes. If you ask me how I am and I tell the truth, I usually get a look of panic from the other person. A look of oh shit, what did I just open and how long do I have to listen before I can exit stage right?? OR I see the look of complete sadness on your face for me and then I put it in reverse to make you feel better, to make you more hopeful for me, to make you believe I am being positive enough about my situation. I realized this after spending some long needed quality time with a great friend. A friend who gets it, a friend who lets me open up all my stuck windows and air out my house. A friend who doesn't look at the trash in my house and tell me if I only did this or that, I wouldn't be in the situation I am in. A friend who accepts what I can and what I can't do. I can go over to her house and hang out for long overdue conversations, but I can't go out to eat for dinner because no matter how little I did that day I am exhausted by 6:00pm. A friend who lets me mourn the loss of the old me without making me feel guilty for being sad with the new me, a me I am still not used to although this me has been here almost two years.

My new me. Yes I am very grateful I am still alive after having Stage IV cancer for three years, many women don't make it this long, but I haven't fully been able to accept my new limitations. My entire right leg is completely numb which makes walking and driving much more of a challenge. I cringe when someone says I need to get out and exercise to help myself heal. They are right, I do. But I don't want to go alone because I am afraid of falling and I don't want to go with anyone because I am so slow I feel bad that I am holding them up. My right arm kind of free floats a lot of the time and I am usually not sure where it is unless I hold it down at my side. I no longer feel comfortable holding any babies. Getting dressed takes me way too long even though I am just putting on workout clothes since nothing else fits me. Not being able to feel my leg or arm, I have to inch up what I am putting on a tiny bit at a time. I cringe when someone says I must be doing so well because of my positive attitude. I often wonder how many people in my life would stick around if I did tell the truth all the time. If I did let this ugly monster out to roam, not just around Eric...what would you say?

My life is a rollercoaster. Not a rollercoaster I ever wanted to ride, but I am on it now and I can't get off. Jill summed it up great; she is with me on my roller coaster, the highs, the lows, the sharp turns, the dark tunnels and boring parts. She understands I can't just get on and off this ride when I want to, but for now I'm stuck here in Cancerland. I guess what I am wanting from this post is understanding and compassion. Understanding that this isn't the person I wanted to be and understanding that this is who I am now. Understanding that this person I am now could change again unbeknownst to you in a blink of an eye...be better or worse. Compassion to me to know I have the best of intentions but my ability to follow through on all of my intentions is not against you, it is just me and right now just me is all I can be.

Empathy – April 1, 2014

I am sad to say I have noticed something in my life lately...a lack of empathy, a lack of empathy on my part to others. I don't think this is a brand new thing which makes me sad. I tend to look at people and their problems in measurement against me and my problems.

When someone is complaining about xyz in their life, I tend to start thinking I wonder what they would do if they were dealing with cancer, a dead leg, migraines, depression and all the other things that seem forever stacked against me. I realized while praying the other day, it isn't their problems versus my problems. It isn't a competition of who wins worst day, week or year. And all too often I tend to do that, in my mind at least. While someone is trying to let go of their problems I am thinking in the back of my mind, yeah like that is a real problem. But it is a real problem to them and I shouldn't be so quick to judge because who am I to judge them and their problems? I don't know what it is like in their life, their life as a whole. I have noticed that all I see of a person's life is a snap shot of a snap shot of maybe a day, or maybe only 1 hour of their day. I put so much stock into this snap shot and think I know the whole story when in reality I don't know it all. I don't want to be like this, to always think my problems trump other problems. I want to learn to look at other people with an empathic heart and know what I see is only a snapshot in time in their life.

The Merry-Go-Round – April 25, 2014

Looking at it from the outside in, it looks magical, painted with deep rich colors that demand attention. It moves with fluid smooth motions. Light dances off of the mirrors and the music is hypnotic. The horses fit my body like glove, like it was carved just me. The excitement builds as I get closer to the entrance, and just as it is my turn to get in the gate and pick my horse, I notice the something different. I can't put my finger on it but I feel it in my soul.

Then there I was, left to pick my horse. I picked a seat bench because if truth be told I am not a huge fun of the up and down motion while going round and round. My seat was hard with a tilted back that made for a comfortable ride. I found myself in awe of the detailed carvings, how does one have the patience for that I wonder to myself? Giggles, laughter and music filled the air, until it didn't.

I was asked to change seats to a whole new ride, to be with a new group of people I didn't know. This seemed normal, like they were my tribe. The air was heavier over here. Like something intense was about to happen and no one looked each other in the eye for fear of the other person seeing this fear too. If they noticed it also, it had to be true, right? I started to notice cracks in the paint and splinters on the pole and sad eyes all around. I asked where we were at, but nobody answered, nobody knew. We would sometimes stop and pick up a few new people or drop someone off. I wanted off. How were they getting off? Why were they getting off and no one around me got to get off? Then I noticed something. Once they got off, they never got back on, we never got to see them again. They just kind of floated into the air all the while we were left there to wonder. So as tired as I was going up and down and round and round, I told myself I had to settle in and try to enjoy the ride.

Then an amazing thing happened, those of us who were left on the ride noticed each other. Noticed we weren't alone on the ride. Noticed there were more things we had in common with one another than being stuck on this ride trying to get off. We noticed all of our horses or bench seats were different in major and minor ways. They all had a different story to tell, once we stopped to listen to each other. We asked why. Why was everyone so different but so much the same? No one knew the answer though. All we knew was that someone heard once you made it to this ride; you were going to be on this ride for the rest of your life. That shook us all to the core. Who said that? How did they know? We all looked at each other so scared we couldn't talk. We just cried.

After all the tears dried up, we all had this magical glow around us. We realized we were there, there for each other, there to help a new one on to the ride; although we really hated it. But we were there none the less for each other, no matter how long or short someone had been on the ride. We were there. There to cry together, to laugh together, to live this life on this merry go round together. We also realized none of us asked for this. None of us did or didn't do one little thing that made us end up here, we were just here.

It made it a little easier to know someone else knew what this fucking ride felt like. We talked with each other. We got to know each other. We asked each other questions. What we did before we were on this ride? What is your family like? Where is your favorite place to be? What are you scared of? That was the one that always got us all. What were we scared of? None of us could help it, that question would take our breath away and made our hearts race. We were scared of dying in our 30's, our kids not having moms, and so much more. We are scared we didn't do enough to have our legacy live on? How will we ever know?

Just a day – April 28, 2014

The air had been thick with heat, humidity and wonder all day. I tried not to let thoughts of yesterday's PET scan slip into my mind, but those thoughts seemed to find any crack and so easily slip in and take over. Today was scheduled as an off day, at least on the books it was. I didn't have treatment today but I had my scan yesterday and waiting for the results was no day at the beach. But I guess in my world there really was never a true off day, especially for my mind.

As I sat there, my stomach churned from the lunch I just ate with

my girlfriends. It wasn't even much food, but I didn't think it was
the food making my stomach hurt. I didn't seem to be able to
eat much in one sitting those days. You would think I could lose
weight eating these smaller meals, I couldn't. My head had a
slight headache from the one cocktail I nursed at lunch and from
the many, many laughs I shared with my girls. My feet and hands
were already beginning to swell from the food and drink. I often
wondered why I swelled so easily and if it had anything to do with
me getting cancer? I guess I will never know. But it was worth it.
Lunch with the girls was always worth it, even if I was laid up for a
day or two after it from using every ounce of my energy and more.
I felt like a wet rag wrung out and ran through the ringer. You know
those ones at the self-serve carwash that would get every last drop
of water out of the rag?

I needed this time with them to feel a tad normal again. Something
I had not felt in a long time and actually wondered if it was
possible for me to feel again. Lunch with them used to be at least
a two to three times a week outing. We would gather those of us
who could go out of the five of us mommies and our kids and go
wherever our hearts desired. We would take the kids to bounce
houses, playgrounds, museums, just us and our kids. We felt like
we could take on the world with our group. Life seemed so simple
and pure back then. We would laugh until we cried. We never ran
out of stuff to talk about. We never thought those days would end.
The kids loved having each other to play with. Sure we would have
to break up a fight here and there, we would wipe the tears after a
fall, and we would carry the kids from the car after they fell asleep
on the way home.

That was my life with them, with my mommy friends. But that was
then, this is now. It is a hard realization to come to, that those days
are gone in so many ways. The kids have school, others have had
other babies, and I will always have on-going cancer treatment.
It may not always kick my ass like this, but it may. Only time

will tell. I can never know how I am going to feel one day to the next. My head might feel like a balloon about to pop from all the pressure on the inside and I sleep away two to three days with no recollection of what happened during those days. Some days my head doesn't hurt, but my heart feels like it is crumbling due to the anxiety I feel about all of this. The anxiety about my life spinning out of control and I just have to sit back and watch. Some days I feel good enough to fake it. Fake it to myself and others that this will all be okay. I can almost fake it until I start to believe it, believe this is all one big ugly dream. But, I always wake up.

On the edge – May 8, 2014

I feel that I am on an edge.

An edge I have been on too many times. An edge I am all too familiar with.

An edge that is exhilarating and completely exhausting...all at the same time.

An edge I can't seem to get away from. An edge I have crossed too many times, both climbing over it and falling off it. Since this thing called cancer entered my life back in 2008, I seem to live on this edge. It seems that I am always on one side of the edge. It is either all or nothing. I can't walk the middle ground. My current edge is my health, which seems to be the theme of most of my edges the past 6 years. Either physical or mental health, or both. Since December of last year I have been standing on this particular edge, waiting...wishing...praying. I just want to be on one side or the other. I want to either feel good or feel like shit for an extended period of time. And yes I realize how weird that sounds, but this up and down cycle I continue to go through is starting to get the best of me. I never know what is next, what the next day holds for me... will I be able to walk without a cane, will my head hurt so bad all I can do is sleep, will I be dizzy and nauseated, will I be able to drive, will I feel like talking on the phone, will I want to write or paint. What does my tomorrow hold for me? I never know until I am there. And all that living in the moment stuff is great and all, but really, I am tired of living in the moment because for once I would like to plan out a little of my life.

We had a scheduled cruise to leave on Easter Sunday with Eric's family. I was so looking forward to that cruise, to just be. To get out of the house and pretend I felt great. But, we didn't get to go. I started having migraines again (or whatever you want to call them). My necrosis was swelling again. I could barely walk. I was sleeping 15ish hours a day. I was a mess in every possible way. It was like it was in December when they decided it was necrosis, but this time felt more intense. Maybe because I was already so worn down it felt more intense or maybe it actually was?

Is this my life now, a series of cycles like this? I don't want to think that, but it is too hard not to. A week of hell with mind numbing headaches, a week of getting back on my feet, a week of being on my feet, only to start the cycle all over again? Doesn't sound like the life I thought I had bartered with God for.

After starting back on the necrosis eating chemo, my fourth round was just like my first. I thought my head was once again going to explode and I wasn't sure I could handle the pain any longer. I had debilitating headaches, I couldn't walk without help, I couldn't drive, I couldn't think clearly and I was falling deeper and deeper into my dark hole.

I prayed, I prayed hard that God would get on with whatever He was going to do. If He was going to fix me I wanted Him to please do it. I was at the end of my rope and needed that fixing soon. I hurt more than I knew I could hurt. The necrosis eating pain was different from the necrosis growing pain. The eating pain completely took me out. I slept for three days straight only waking up a few times to eat or use the restroom. I didn't remember it being this bad the very first time, but Eric assured me it was. Not only did my head, neck, and shoulders hurt, but my heart hurt. My heart hurt because I was sure me and God had made a deal. I promised to write more of my story to help others and He promised to keep the pain away. That was my deal at least. I guess looking back He never agreed to that deal. But here I am today, three days out from necrosis eating chemo #5 and feeling pretty good. I have a headache and get queasy if I move my head too fast or am in the car. Every day that goes by, I get further and further from the scary side of the ledge and creep closer and closer to the middle, where I pray I stay for long, long time.

My Color Bomb– May 12, 2014

I can say it. I can finally say it and truly mean it. I feel it in my soul, my way down deep soul. My way down deep soul that has been praying and dreaming about this for so long. I felt my soul blowing out the grey clouds that have been clinging on to me for life support the past six months. These grey clouds seemed to penetrate every part of my body, but the place I felt it most was my heart. It seemed I would see a break in the clouds for a short time, only for them to roll back in for a full on thunderstorm that would never release rain. The threat of the storm hung in the air for everyone to feel, not just me. My heart has been so many things but at peace these last six months. I have had this unsettling turmoil swirling through my mind and body. I imagine this turmoil to look like a child's drawing. A child who secretly stole a pack of crayons and colored a picture on the walls, fast and furious. Not intending to hurt anything or anyone...he just had the urge to do it. A picture of nothing but messy scribbles at first glance, s picture of chaos, like a color bomb exploded. No matter what way I turned the picture, I couldn't find anything in the chaos, especially beauty. I almost gave up looking at my color bomb. I so wanted to crumble it up and toss it in the trash can. But just as I began to crumble it up, the color boom showed me something. It showed me the layers and layers that I had to put into this picture to get it to look like it does.

It was a picture of my life...of all life. It isn't what we see on the surface that makes the picture have depth and meaning, it is all the layers dropped on each other. This weekend was just another layer added to my picture of life. It was a beautiful layer, full of moments I wasn't really ever sure I would get to experience again. I went to Ian's soccer game and I was there. I was really there, in the moment, cheering the team on and enjoying the noise and chaos. We went to an end of year party, and I was there too. Not my shell that I have been totting around with me, it was me there. I socialized with new people, I held up my end of conversations, I was me. The old me who I really thought had been eatin' up by cancer and necrosis.

I painted again!

I painted from my heart.

I painted from that place that makes me giddy with delight.

I painted with bright colors that made my soul smile. A smile that hasn't been seen in way too long.

This weekend made me finally realize that yes my life has changed so much since I started this cancer journey, but it is just one more layer to add to my picture.

So what if life is completely different from when I didn't have cancer. I do have it now and always will. I just need to always remember to look at my color bomb and find one little corner of beauty and the rest will come.

My 36th year?!?! – May 13, 2014

Last year I wasn't really sure I would live to see my 36th birthday. My 35th year was full of ups and downs. I just didn't know…I honestly didn't know if I had more fight in me to get me through anymore. I was told a few days before I turned 35 that my brain tumor was back for the third time. I was just getting back to life and then there it was again ready to try to take me down. That tumor has been my cruise director for the past 20 months. It has dictated what I could and couldn't do both mentally and physically. It sided more with what I couldn't do. I am afraid if I list all my moments, both good and bad, and line the lists up side by side, the down side would be much, much longer than the up side. That is hard to stomach. But when I do look on the good side of the list, I see many important points.

I am still alive asshole tumor

Only one brain surgery!

I can drive again

Learning to reenter society, my society I have missed so much

Wanting to paint and write

Yeah, just one brain operation and 3 brain radiations compared to the year before!?!?!

I lost count of radiations. It makes my heart hurt and so happy all at the same time just thinking about it. Knowing all the pain and uncertainty this past year held for me and Eric and all our loved ones. It was a tough year. I feel good about this year though feel more connected to my soul. I am working on forgiveness, forgiveness to God, to myself, to my situation. Through much journaling and some hard questions to my soul, I realized I was holding on to a lot of resentment. Resentment for all this that I have viewed as unfair, but I have come to realize God never

promised fair. He just promised to get me through it. I started
physical therapy this week. I know it will get me moving which
will help in the long run even though it is hard as hell right now.
Painting for the sheer joy of painting, it really feels like I could see
light from my heart shining onto the painting. I have fully decided
and have actually started (don't be too shocked!) to turn this blog
into a book?!?! I have been going back through all my old entries
and adding more emotion and detail. It is funny how easy I can go
back to that place when I read the old entries. And today I found
out one more piece of news that has solidified the fact that the
best is yet to come.

Drum roll pleas...My whole body is cancer free!!!!!! A head and
full body PET scan showed it...no hot spots to be found. Thank you
God! Thank you all for all of your prayers, support and love. I can't
wait to see what is next for us! Maybe we will finally get to take
that vacation?!

The Ribbon – May 22, 2014

A twirling ribbon dances in the sky

Taken up by a gust of wind –

Not to make anyone sad for losing it

But to make everyone around stop what they are doing take notice

It looks as if God is playing with us from the sky

We are His young children being entertained

*By this ribbon that dances in the sky so delicately it does a loop-de-
loop*

I hold my breath not knowing if it will make it all the way around

But it does make it around

Only to go on and perform a back and forth dance with the breeze

With God it creates big beautiful waves riding on the air

Like a skilled surfer dancing on the waves

I couldn't help but feel the wonder build

Dreaming of what it will do next

I can't see the air making this ribbon dance

But I am fully aware of the light cool breeze

It blows on my face through the otherwise warm air

Then all of a sudden all is still

And the ribbon floats back towards the ground With grace

With delight it floats to me and lands softly in my lap

I look around to see if anyone else is going to claim it

But it seems it was dropped here for me

From God as a reminder

He is always here

He is always here

It hurts so bad – June 9, 2014

Well, all my "oh, this chemo is a breeze" is coming back to bite me or burn me I should say. I am experiencing a very common side effect of this chemo called hand-foot syndrome Let me tell you, this crap hurts. Me feet hurt the worse, especially when I am on them...so my grand plan to start walking to lose weight is once again put on hold. Can't I just live my life Sorry the pictures are gross, but my feet are gross and in pain. The bottoms feel sunburnt and swollen. And my hands are so tender bending them hurt. Cream helped a bit when it first started, but not now. I guess another day in Cancerland

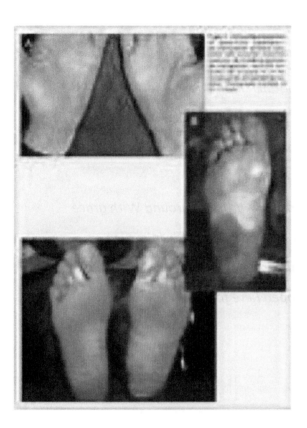

Therapy – June 12, 2014

At one point in my life, I would never write this. I used to be embarrassed that I needed therapy of any kind. I used to think I should be able to handle all this on my. I used to think a lot of things that I look back on and think, wow that is so stupid. Honestly, I never knew one person could see so many different therapists at the same time. When people ask me what I do all day, I am so temped to say, "Therapy, that is the long and short of it."

Seriously though here is a list of what I do:

Chemotherapy: Well you know, for that cancer bit and stuff. I go for infusion once every third week, and I take six chemo pills at home for two weeks on and one week off. So really I am on chemo about 70% of the time.

Head therapy: Dr. H told me a few weeks ago that it was that time once again, to pick up my pieces and start moving forward. I feel like a pack mule hauling all of my issues around. She asked me if I ever went back to the therapist who she told me to go to. I told her I went four times and she looked at me with that mom look of *really?!* She said that isn't good enough. I need to KEEP going. She likes to remind me I have been dealing with cancer in some form for the past six years and four therapy sessions isn't going to work it all out. I was prone to depression before all this started six years ago. I guess chemo didn't take that away for me. So now I do talk therapy once a week.

Physical therapy: Again, Dr. H was all up in my business about this too and told me it was time to go back. I fought her on this for a long time too. I didn't want to go back. It is hard. It makes me tired. It makes me sad, sad to see what I am not able to do anymore. It pisses me off. Going there and having to learn how to walk again for the third time now. It isn't something that I want to admit I need help with. Relearning how to walk, balance, gain strength back, avoid falls and so much more is so hard. It is hard physically and emotionally. I mean, I used to be able to do so much and then one day I couldn't, repeat times three.

Hypnotherapy: She didn't tell me to do this, I just do it on my own. I quit smoking about 10 years ago with hypnosis and I have never smoked again. So to say the least, I am a big believer in it. Eric thinks it is BS, but I think it depends on the person. I tell him he just thinks he is too smart for it and roll my eyes at him. I started back with hypnosis a few months for my anxiety, depression, confidence and any other lingering issues that seem to like to hang around. I love it. I know this doesn't replace my talk therapy and my meds that I am on for depression and anxiety, but I like it. If nothing else to help me relax for an hour.

Family and Friend Therapy: I am getting out again, learning to be social again. I am learning to lean on others and not just Eric all the time. I am learning to trust my words that I tell so many others. People want to help and want to feel needed.

Creative Therapy: I am writing more than ever. I can officially say I have started my book of this journey I have been on these past six years. I am painting again. I am learning to live again. Live my life as I am now.

Once bitten, twice shy – June 17, 2014

That is how I feel now in regards to scans. I had a head MRI on Friday, saw Dr. H and had two chemos yesterday, and went to Groves to look at my MRI from Friday. To say the least, I am beat down tired today with a headache from the chemo and just being so tired. But I will take it because I am still NED in my head and in my body. Oh it is that little things NED that make my heart happy! Yes, I realize it isn't little!

I got a little lecture from Dr. H yesterday when I told her what all I had been doing. She told me to slow my roll. We just laugh together.

Infusion was easy, then I came home and half slept half listened for my alarm to go off to tell me it was time to go to Groves. Eric went with me downtown because I still don't feel comfortable driving downtown and man I am glad he was with me. After a long wait (which I don't mind with Groves, you can't rush a genius in my opinion), we talked to Dr. Groves; he said my MRI looks better and better every time and we will just keep this train rolling. I got my next MRI pushed out for 10 weeks which is great! He said of course call if need be earlier, but honestly he doesn't want to see me earlier. And I him! I am tired today after yesterday having two treatments and all the appointments, so I am going to sit it on the couch today and do nothing. See, I am learning to listen to my body. Maybe I should send this to Dr. H?!?!

Two headed monster – July 21, 2014

Back in 2010, I was diagnosed with depression and put on medicine. I chose not to write about it then because I was afraid to admit it.

I saw it as a sign of weakness.

Guess what?

It didn't just go away. It needs to be talked about and now I can look back and say it's nothing to be ashamed of.

I don't know if I have come out and said it before, but I struggle with depression and anxiety. Once we got home from our trip, the two headed monster came for me. Some days I do good telling it where to stick it. Other days, the monster scares me into submission. It gets in my head and makes up this whole long movie about what a loser I am for not being able to do more…like my other cancer friends do. Or if the monster is feeling really dirty it will make me believe the cancer is back, slowly eating my brain again. I know, it sounds like a page out of a horror book, but this is my truth. Eric told me I needed to write more because he can tell a difference in me when I write and just get it out. I figure y'all are sick of hearing about this crap. Again, the monster talking. But I do feel better getting it out of me. Telling the world (or whoever reads this?) my truth. I want to start telling my truth all the time.

Then what – July 23, 2014

I went to see the movie Boyhood this weekend with a dear friend I don't get to see often because life is busy.

This movie touched me way down deep, the deep that makes me get all giddy because I see that other people think the same as I do. I have been holding out for the WOW moment in my life. Even with cancer, I have been holding out for something, for the next something to be wowed at.

At first, I was waiting for the cancer to be gone. Then it was (the first time). Then I was waiting to be like I was before cancer, then I was. Then I got cancer again. Then I was waiting until it was gone, then it was. Then it wasn't.

In between all these huge moments that make up this life, I too easily forget that it is in between these huge moments...that is real life. Yes, I have more peaks and valleys then most people, but I am really trying harder to enjoy the whole ride, not just the breathing-taking drops, and being ok with the mundane coasting. I am finding out, that is where you see all the pretty scenery.

The Fight – July 24, 2014

The air is thick with excitement from the on-lookers ready to see someone go down. They are ready to see someone get punched with an iron fist and get laid out flat. Not a real iron fist of course, but a fist so strong it feels like metal is hidden somewhere in that glove. The crowd is getting fired up as the seconds from the clock tick away. Tick away to where, no one really knows or cares. Then just like that, it is here. Fight time is here. The fighters are introduced one at a time. A hush so intense falls over the crowd.

You can hear the metallic cloth rubbing together of the fighter's shorts as she walks into the ring. You can see the sweat glisten on her body as the fighter steps in and out of the spotlight.

"In this corner, we have the defending champion" blares out of the speakers. She is adorned with gold from head to toe and has a look in her eye that scares even the on-lookers who are thanking God right now that it isn't them who must fight this beast. "And in the other corner, we have a newbie here at the ring. She comes to us from Austin, with no prior training in this field of fighting. Our surprise guest is such a surprise, she doesn't even know she will be fighting until right at this moment. Renee, come on down."

I look around to see who else is named Renee. How bizarre I think to myself. Why would they make a surprise guest fight? Then I notice that no one stands up. You can feel the crowd getting more inpatient by the second as everyone's anxiety starts to grow. The spot light is now shinning its harsh light into my eyes. I put my arm up to shield the direct beam assault. My heart jumps into my throat as I think to myself this is a cruel joke to be playing on me. Don't these people know my right leg is numb from one too many brain surgeries? Don't these people know I have had cancer one too many times? Don't these people care? All eyes are on me now. The crowd goes quiet, just looking at me. Just waiting to see what I will do. I don't know what to do.

Then I hear it from deep in my heart whispering to me that I have to do this. This whisper tells me I will be ok, more than ok. I will be great. I tell my heart I don't want to. I don't want to go. I didn't sign up for this shit. Someone else signed up for it, not me. There it is again, my name being called out over the loud booming speaker that echoes off the walls and around in my head. The intense stares from the crowd are starting to eat into my soul. I know I can't get out of this. I don't know how I got into this, but I know

I can't walk away from it. These people came to see a fight and they won't leave until they do. Somewhere, somehow I am now walking up to the ring. I guess to fight, but to tell the truth I have no idea. I don't feel myself thinking about walking, my feet are just moving. I have never fought before. I have never hit someone nor had someone hit me. How is this happening to me, keeps running through my head.

Then there I am looking at myself like I am looking in a full-length mirror, but there is a shine in my eye I have never noticed before. I am not sure who is who. Who am I? Am I in the mirror? Am I in the ring? The announcer tells us to shake on a fair fight as he grabs our hands to reach them out to touch one another in the middle. It takes all I have not pull my hand back to my side. All I can think at this point is the sooner this starts, the sooner it will be over. I try to yell out, that it is me. Both of the fighters are me. No one seems to notice, or care. We do some fancy foot work around each other for what seems like eternity. I hear a voice from the crowd yell out, "do it! Hit her!" I wanted to look at who was yelling this but I knew I couldn't look away. I held my breath, locked eyes with myself and sent my fist flying through the air with a force I didn't know I had in me. Then that was it.

The mirror image of me stepped towards me and hugged me. One of the tightest, whole hearted hugs I have ever felt. Every ounce of guilt, anger, judgment and all the black ick I had held over my own head for all my life came crumbling down. Once I realized what was happening, that I was reaching into hug myself, I crumbled into me. I realized that I was forgiving myself for all that had happened in my life. For all that I have blamed myself for all these years. For all the guilt I have lugged around with me for too long. Then, I heard it again. That voice, that voice that was so kind and gentle it was almost magical. It said, "I knew you could do it. All you had to do was believe in yourself as much as others do."

Enough – July 31, 2014

All around me, I see people doing so much more than I am able to. More work, more working out, more volunteering, more cooking, more cleaning...the list could go on forever. It is hard for me not to beat myself up about this, tell myself that I should be able to do more, I should be able to volunteer more, make videos more, create more artwork, more, more, more. But I can't. I just can't if I want to be the person I want to be so much. I have to realize I am doing all I can, all I need to do and I am doing enough. I am enough.

Letter to Ian – August 11, 2014

Dear Ian,

Seven years old. Oh my sweet little guy. You aren't so little anymore. You are the tallest in your class and nobody believes me when I tell them you are not eight or nine. You have grown up so much this past year. You loved Kindergarten, won the Excellent Award for being a great listener, helper and classmate. We are so proud to see you growing into a caring human being. Anytime we see anyone in need, you want to know what you can do to help. You ask me to stop at every homeless person we see to give them money. You question why people are mean to others. You question why others lie. Your heart is honest and pure. Me and daddy tell you that even when others are mean or lie, you need to love them anyway because we don't know what is happening in their life that we don't see. You 100% take that to heart. You tell me if someone was mean to someone else at school or camp that you hope they are both ok. You are truly a beacon of light in this world.

We got Lucy this year. You love to lay in her bed with her and let her lick your face. She is still a little nippy, so you are still learning how to play fetch with her. You are developing your own unique sense of humor. You are very dry and matter of fact with what you say, but the grin on your face makes everyone laugh. You still love to make me and daddy laugh. You love anything to do with science, you want to read non-fiction fact books about dinosaurs and rocks, you have figured out how to win big at Chucky Cheese with BeBe's help in counting when the wheel will stop on the grand prize. You and BeBe have people ask for help in winning the jackpot all the time when we are there. You went to summer camp in the neighborhood this summer and had a great time. You also went to Lego camp and have become a great builder. You still love Pokemon and love your collection of them. I love you more than words could ever explain. You have a piece of my heart that makes me, you and daddy a complete whole.

I love you so much

A messy puddle – August 17, 2014

Man oh man; I am ready for summer to be over. It is flipping hot here and me plus hot equals beat down Renee. When I get beat down, I crumble. I crumble too easily. I crumbled this weekend. I am not really sure why, but I did. I crumbled into a puddle. That puddle led me to a panic attack that led to guilt that led to uck. I am tired of crumbling. I do wonder if I will ever stop crumbling or if I will continue to crumble but learn how to deal with it?

For a reason – August 22, 2014

I had a PET scan and MRI scheduled today for about two weeks now. They were scheduled to be back to back because going multiple times is a pain in the ass. But I got a call yesterday asking me if I would mind if they pushed my PET to an hour later. I said sure, no problem. I knew I would be starving, but other than not being able to eat, I had nothing else going on today. After my MRI, I went to another waiting area to wait for my PET scan. I had all my shit spread out as usual because I was planning on camping out there to work on Renee In Cancerland stuff. My plans changed quickly as soon as I watched a scared mother walk in with her daughter to sit and wait also. I heard that famous whisper talking to my heart and I did what it told me to do, even at the sake of looking like a crazy person, nothing too new to me! My heart told me to talk to them. So I walked over, pulled up a chair, asked them if I could sit. I asked them what was going on. The mom told me her daughter was there for a PET scan, that she was just diagnosed and a PET is the first step to see if the cancer is elsewhere. I reached out to hold their hands. I looked at her and her daughter in the eyes and told them that this sucks. Plain and simple, this sucks. Then I explained a little of my story, because lets me honest, no one who is just diagnosed really wants to hear all my crap. I told her it is ok to be scared, it is ok to be pissed, it is ok to not want to be brave, it is ok to want to run and hide...all that is ok.

BUT then you have to look up at whatever it is, look it in the eyes and tell it to eat shit. They laughed. It made my heart happy. She was called back before me, so I sat out in the waiting area. I was talking with the lady at the front desk and she said thank you to me for what I did for them. She told me that she sees so many people who wouldn't have taken those unknown steps, and she was grateful I was there and I did. I left all my contact info with her and asked her to give it to her mother on their way out. I asked her to PLEASE tell the mom to call me because I am serious about talking to her and her daughter...it wasn't just an empty offer. Then

I was called back to get injected with my nuclear sugar water. The mom and daughter were back there waiting for her PET to start. She wanted to take a picture with me. I was honored. Then Fred told me I had to stop roaming around and go sit down to let my nuclear stuff do what it needed to. I left there feeling good. I left there knowing God had changed my appointment so I could be there for them. I left there with a little pep in my step knowing it really did matter, it really did help them. My Bible verse from this morning was: Guard your heart above all else, for it determines the course of your life. Proverbs 4:23

PET scan and MRI results – August 27, 2014

So sorry I forgot to post the results here. I am still NED (no evidence of disease) in my body!!!! There was a slight change in my brain MRI, BUT Dr. H thinks it is due to the Avastin (the necrosis eating chemo). I go see Groves (brain oncologist) on the 8th. My guess is all is well since no one has called to change my appointment, if something was bad they would move my appointment up. SO, we will go with the nothing new assumption for now!

Feathers from Angels – August 30, 2014

Feathers from Angels I have been trying to take notice of the little things around me, the little things that have always been there but sometimes I was too preoccupied with myself to notice. Too preoccupied with what I was worrying about. Too preoccupied with what I thought others were thinking. Too preoccupied comparing myself to myself of the past, the me who could do so much more. I took a class on how to hear your angels, as I believe God gives us all angels to be with us all the time. And no, I don't think it is because God can't do it all, it is because He has people with Him who are born to help others. And they still want to help others no matter if they are on earth or not. From this class, so much came rushing back to me, so many memories that I had forgotten about: Times where there is NO explanation of how it worked out so beautifully. Times where I follow that feeling of guidance and it lead me to a magical place. Times where I cry out for help only to look around and see He has already sent help. With all my prayer work lately, I have felt the nudge to call for help in all I do. And I mean ALL, even the tiny things that seem to not matter. From this, I have been noticing magic all around me. Call it what you would like, I call it friendship from above. Like God is our father sending out an older sibling to watch me and make sure I am ok. I now see fresh fluffy feathers all throughout the day. When I wake up, there is a feather in the restroom. When I leave the house, there is a feather on the front doorstep. When I get in the car, there is a feather on my windshield. With these little tokens from above, I tell God thank you for sending Angels. I tell the Angels thank you for being with me.

Wrapping it up - September 8, 2014

It is a bright sunny Monday morning. I am sitting in my writing chair in disbelief that I am on the closing chapter of this book. Before sitting down to write this morning, I got up with Ian and played with him before school, rode my motorized trike over to Gina's for much needed friend time and did a meditation.

So, if you are wondering how I am now I can honestly say great... fantastic! I don't always feel great. In fact just a few days ago I was in my pajamas for three days straight because I had been way over doing it for too long. I crashed. I crashed hard. My body couldn't do anymore. So no, I have not learned where that line is between just enough and too much. I still cross over it and regret it and say I won't ever do that again. I am pretty sure I will though.

It is like drinking a little too much one night, waking up feeling like crap the next day, swearing to never do it again but then months later you are with your people and it just happens. Good times just happen. As far as my treatment goes, I take oral chemo daily and get an infusion once every three weeks; the oral chemo kind of sucks. I am always constipated and it dries my feet and hands out so bad they crack. I have found if I use Ava Anderson products a few times a day I can kind of combat this but not entirely. I haven't found a way around the constipation. I eat veggies, six to eight servings per day and fruits two to three serving per day and am still having issues.

I get a PET scan and brain MRI every three months, AND the last one, which was two weeks ago still showed NED...yes NED in both head and body!!! So, I guess technically you can say I am cancer free right at this moment in time!!

We went to church for the first time yesterday in almost two years. To say it was wonderful would be an understatement. I felt like the missing piece to my soul was put back in.

I have started doing art again! People are loving my Cancer Girl paintings and just general feel good statement pieces. I am working on finding a place to print them so I can share them with more people.

I have prayed for so long that my art would somehow change the world, I believe it can and it will.

I have plans to contact all the hospitals/treatment centers/ magazines/etc who used my scarf picture to tell them about this book and ask for help getting it out! "Why not"? That is my to-slogan these days.

Eric is doing great. We are talking about getting a conversion van to travel being as air travel and me don't get along too well.

Ian is in first grade, plays soccer, has great friends (yes, he is just like me when it comes to making new friends!) and is just an all-around great kid. We talk about my cancer when he wants to, he sometimes asks me when I feel good for a long period of time if I am still sick. He will ask me when I am super tired if it is because of the cancer. Unfortunately he has seen me have a few panic attacks and I see the fear in his eyes. But no matter what, Eric and I always tell him the truth.

I don't want to leave you hanging by not wrapping this up, but for right now, it is wrapped up. I really hope to never have another "adventure" like this to write a book about again, but I will promise you this: This isn't the last time you will hear from me. I still have a lot of work to do for God in this world, I plan to change it one heart at a time.

With love,

Renee

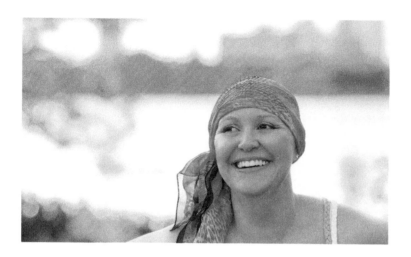

RENEE SENDELBECH

First diagnosed with Stage 1 breast cancer at the young age of 30 when her son was only 13 months old, Renee has been through more in 6 years than most go through in a life time.

Countless chemotherapies, breast and brain radiation, three brain surgeries and so much more, Renee writes from her heart about her highest ups and lowest lows in a refreshingly honest voice.

There is no sugarcoating the hardships here, but there is a hope that can be found throughout all of her struggles. She writes like she is sitting with you telling you the story with all the witty lines she says in her day-to-day life.

This book isn't just for others with breast cancer. This book is for all who hold onto hope at every turn in life.

Renee resides in Austin, Texas with her husband Eric, son, Ian and Lucy, the family dog who drives her nuts!

CPSIA information can be obtained at www.ICGtesting.com
Printed in the USA
BVOW10s1312170715

408911BV00010B/65/P